DANCE/MOVEMENT
THERAPISTS IN ACTION

ABOUT THE EDITORS

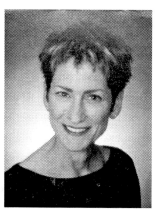

ROBYN FLAUM CRUZ, PH.D., ADTR, studied dance/movement therapy at New York University, and received her doctorate in educational psychology specializing in measurement and methodology from The University of Arizona. Her work as a methodologist has spanned quantitative and qualitative research in many fields including dance/movement therapy, psychology, psychiatry, and neurology. Her work has been published in professional journals such as, *Brain, Neuropsychologia, Psychiatric Services, Archives of Neurology*, and *American Journal of Dance Therapy*. She was co-editor of the *American Journal of Dance Therapy* from 1998 to 2001. She is Director of Creative and Expressive Arts Therapies at Western Psychiatric Institute and Clinic of the University of Pittsburgh Medical Center, Pittsburgh, PA, and Editor-in-Chief of *The Arts in Psychotherapy*.

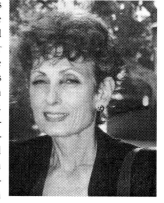

CYNTHIA F. BERROL, PH.D., ADTR, is Professor Emerita of California State University, Hayward, where she developed and co-directed the former Special Graduate Major in Dance/Movement Therapy (DMT). She received her M.A. degree in dance from Mills College and her doctorate in special education from the University of California, Berkeley. Dr. Berrol has authored a range of articles—theoretical, clinical, and research based—addressing DMT, and has lectured and consulted nationally and internationally. In 1987, as an invited consultant, she piloted a dance/movement therapy program at the Rehabilitation Center for Brain Damage at the University of Copenhagen, Denmark. Currently, she serves on the editorial boards of three professional journals.

DANCE/MOVEMENT THERAPISTS IN ACTION

A Working Guide to Research Options

By

ROBYN FLAUM CRUZ

and

CYNTHIA F. BERROL

With a Foreword by

JOAN CHODOROW

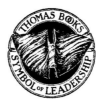

CHARLES C THOMAS • PUBLISHER, LTD.
Springfield • Illinois • U.S.A.

Published and Distributed Throughout the World by

CHARLES C THOMAS • PUBLISHER, LTD.
2600 South First Street
Springfield, Illinois 62704

© 2004 by CHARLES C THOMAS • PUBLISHER, LTD

ISBN 0-398-07504-2 (hard)
ISBN 0-398-07505-0 (paper)

Library of Congress Catalog Card Number: 2004044071

Printed in the United States of America
JW-R-3

Library of Congress Cataloging-in-Publication Data

Cruz, Robyn Flaum.
    Dance/movement therapists in action : a working guide to research options
/ by Robyn Flaum Cruz and Cynthia F. Berrol ; with a foreword by Joan
Chodorow.
        p. cm.
    Includes bibliographical references and index.
    ISBN 0-398-07504-2 — ISBN 0-398-07505-0 (pbk.)
        1. Dance therapy—Research—Methodology.   2. Movement therapy—
Research—Methodology.   I. Berrol, Cynthia Florence.   II. Title.

RC489.D3C78 2004
615.8'5155—dc22

                                                                                2004044071

CONTRIBUTORS

Cynthia F. Berrol, Ph.D., ADTR, Professor Emerita, California State University, Hayward (CSUH) developed and coordinated the former Special Graduate major in Dance/Movement Therapy at CSUH, and has lectured and consulted nationally and internationally. She has authored numerous dance/movement therapy related articles and is on the editorial boards of *Journal of Head Trauma Rehabilitation, American Journal of Dance Therapy,* and *The Arts in Psychotherapy.* She served as treasurer of the American Dance Therapy Association for four years. She remains an active member of the Research Committee of the American Dance Therapy Association, which she chaired for four years. She was Project Associate of the ADTA Demonstration Project studying the effects of DMT on older individuals with brain injuries and stroke, funded by the Administration on Aging of the Department of Health and Human Services.

Harris Chaiklin, Ph.D., is Professor Emeritus at the University of Maryland School of Social Work. As a member of a professional school faculty he combined practice, teaching, and research. His teaching specialties centered around the social aspects of practice and research. He has special interests in the creative aspects of practice. He has edited the papers of Marian Chace and has published articles on the need for research by dance therapists.

Sharon Chaiklin, ADTR, is a founding member of the American Dance Therapy Association and was its second president. Trained by Marian Chace, she has had a long career as a practitioner, mainly in psychiatric hospital settings and private practice. She has published several articles and has taught at Goucher College and internationally in Israel, Japan, Korea, and Argentina. Currently she serves as a trustee of the Marian Chace Foundation and continues to be active as a dance performer, appearing at times with The Liz Lerman Dance Exchange.

Robyn Flaum Cruz, Ph.D., ADTR, has taught research design and statistics to students from many disciplines, including dance/movement therapy, at The University of Arizona, New York University, Pratt Institute, and the Rotterdamse Dansacademie in the Netherlands. She served as research and statistical consultant to the National Center for Neurogenic Communication Disorders, Department of Speech and Hearing Sciences, The University of Arizona from 1994 to 1998, and as Director of Research for COPE Behavioral Services, Tucson, Arizona, from 1999 to 2002. She was co-editor of the *American Journal of Dance Therapy* from 1998 to 2001. Dr.

Cruz has been a member of the Research Committee of the American Dance Therapy Association since 1994. In 2002, Dr. Cruz became Director of Creative and Expressive Arts Therapies at Western Psychiatric Institute and Clinic of the University of Pittsburgh Medical Center and Editor-in-Chief of *The Arts in Psychotherapy.*

Michele Forinash, D.A., MT-BC, LMHC, is Associate Professor and acting Co-director of the Expressive Therapies Division at Lesley University, Cambridge, Massachusetts, and Coordinator for music therapy. She received her doctorate in music therapy from New York University. She is currently President of the American Music Therapy Association (www.musictherapy.org). Forinash is the editor of *Music Therapy Supervision* (Barcelona Publishers) and co-editor of *Educators, Therapists, and Artists on Reflective Practice* (Peter Lang Publishers). She has presented in Israel, Norway, England, and Germany, and her publications include articles and chapters on supervision and qualitative research. She is the North American Editor for the online international music therapy journal *Voices: A World Forum for Music Therapy* (www.voices.no).

Sherry W. Goodill, Ph.D., ADTR, LPC, is Associate Professor and Director of Dance/Movement Therapy Education in the Hahnemann Creative Arts in Therapy Program at Drexel University in Philadelphia. She holds a doctorate in medical psychology with a concentration in mind/body studies, and her professional interests are in research, clinical, and training issues in dance/movement therapy. She served on the Board of Directors of the American Dance Therapy Association from 1990 to 2000. She is a member of the dance therapy editorial board for *The Arts in Psychotherapy.*

Jill Green, Ph.D., is Associate Professor of dance at The University of North Carolina at Greensboro. She coordinates the dance education program, conducts research, and teaches dance education and body courses. Dr. Green's research interests include dance education, somatics and body studies, creativity, qualitative research, and feminist research and pedagogy. Her work is published in a number of journals including *Dance Research Journal, Research in Dance Education, Journal of Dance Education, Impulse, Journal of Interdisciplinary Research in Physical Education,* and *Frontiers: A Journal of Women Studies.* Dr. Green has been invited to contribute a number of chapters to dance books. Additionally, she is a Fulbright Scholar and co-editor of *Dance Research Journal.*

Judith Lynne Hanna, Ph.D. (anthropology, Columbia University), is a Senior Research Scholar, Dance Department, University of Maryland, and has conducted field research primarily in Africa and the United Srares. Her books include *Dance and Stress; To Dance Is Human; Dance, Sex, and Gender; The Performer-Audience Connection;* and *Partnering Dance and Education.* Dr. Hanna's nearly three hundred articles in thirteen countries include *American Journal of Dance Therapy* (she has served on the editorial board since 1988) and *Journal of Alternative and Complementary Medicine.* She spoke at the Postgraduate Center for Mental Health, Johns Hopkins University Public Health Program, Uniformed Services University of Health Sciences, School of Medicine, National Symposium on Pain and elsewhere in the United States and abroad.

Lenore Wadsworth Hervey, Ph.D., ADTR, NCC, REAT, holds a doctoral degree from The Union Institute and University in creativity and research. She is a full-time faculty member in the Dance/Movement Therapy Department at Columbia College, Chicago. She was previously a faculty member at Antioch New England Graduate School. Dr. Hervey is the author of *Artistic Inquiry in Dance/Movement Therapy* and co-author of "The ADTA Research Survey." She chairs the Research Committee of the American Dance Therapy Association. She is a registered dance/movement therapist and a registered expressive arts therapist.

Sabine C. Koch, M.S.W., M.A., DTR, BDT, studied psychology at the University of Heidelberg, Germany, and Madrid (UAM), Spain, as well as dance/movement therapy at Hahnemann University in Philadelphia. She has therapy experience with multiple personality disorder patients, autistic children, and geriatric patients. She has specialized in Kestenberg Movement Profiling (KMP), and its use in research and education. Presently she is completing her doctorate in a national research project at the University of Heidelberg (language and social psychology) with micro-analyses of "Communication of Gender and Leadership in Team Meetings." The project focuses on the analysis of verbal and nonverbal interaction patterns and rhythms.

FOREWORD

Robyn Flaum Cruz and Cynthia F. Berrol have produced a book that, like dance therapy itself, fosters awareness of the living body, honors diverse ways of working, and leads toward creative expression and integration. Guided by their vision of a comprehensible and useful text written by authors with exemplary credentials, *Dance/Movement Therapists in Action: A Working Guide to Research Options* is a significant contribution to the literature. This impressive collection of papers offers rich resources to all who contribute to dance therapy practice, education, and scholarship. It is an accessible introduction for students and interns as well as a useful guide for seasoned professionals.

The seeds of this book can be traced to the Research Subcommittee[1] of the American Dance Therapy Association (ADTA). When the committee was established in 1994, Cynthia F. Berrol was appointed its first chair. Then Robyn Flaum Cruz joined and they began their fruitful collaboration. Each brought interest and excitement, as well as rich backgrounds and professional experiences important to research.

As co-editor of the *American Journal of Dance Therapy*, Dr. Cruz invited Dr. Berrol to write a paper that appeared in a special issue devoted to different facets of dance therapy research (Berrol, 2000). From her survey of the literature, it became clear how much writing there was about research in other fields and, by contrast, little about research inquiry in the dance therapy literature. Within the same time frame, Lenore Hervey joined the Research Subcommittee, bringing her innovative perspective on artistic inquiry to dance/movement therapy (Hervey, 2000). As Drs. Berrol, Cruz, and Hervey began to work together, they made the decision to construct a survey of ADTA members to gather information about attitudes, experiences, and needs regarding research. The results of this inquiry (Cruz & Hervey, 2001) reinforced the need for a book directed to dance/movement therapists and provided the impetus to write it. A prospectus submitted to Charles C Thomas was accepted for publication in spring 2002.

This outstanding collection of papers presents a wide range of quantitative and qualitative approaches, encompassing many creative variations. At the same time it is a handbook, offering structures within which creative

---

[1]In October 2000 the American Dance Therapy Association Board of Directors changed the name of the Education Committee, of which research had constituted a subcommittee, to the Education, Research and Practice Committee. Reference in this volume has been shortened to "Research Committee," to reflect the change.

intellect and imagination can flourish. It is such an interesting and engaging book, I found myself holding conversations with it. Just as I ask students to engage scholarly argument with their questions, comments, objections, "what-have-you," I could hardly avoid doing the same thing; not in a polemical sense, but in trying to understand my own preferences and the preferences of others, toward a larger perspective that includes the many ways different individuals make their contribution.

Similar to life itself, research draws from both conscious and unconscious sources. Because every creative process involves an interweaving of consciousness with the unconscious, both realms should be present in every form of research, but at times perhaps, one or the other shifts from background to foreground. Could it be that "objective" approaches emphasize conscious, intentional, ego-directed procedures? By contrast, could it be that "subjective" approaches include procedures that intentionally turn toward the unconscious to evoke creative imagination as well as intellect? I wonder whether some investigators are mainly interested in the answers, while others are mainly interested in the questions?

The closing chapter of this book explores an integrative approach that brings to mind the nature of the opposites, the dynamic tension between them and Jung's early concept of the transcendent function as "a movement out of the suspension between two opposites, a living birth that leads to a new level of being, a new situation" (Jung 1916/1958, p. 90, ¶ 189). In contrasting the paradigm of deductive (quantitative) with inductive (qualitative) research design, Cynthia Berrol draws the analogy to two approaches to movement: "I move" and "I am moved." Pioneer dance therapist Mary Whitehouse described this creative dialectic: "The core of the movement experience is the sensation of moving and being moved. There are many implications in putting it like this. Ideally, both are present in the same instant, and it may literally be an instant. It is a moment of total awareness, the coming together of what I am doing and what is happening to me" (Whitehouse, 1958/1999, p. 43).

We turn now to the valuable contributions that make up this text. Like the research process itself, it is important that these varied approaches be explored and reflected upon by the reader. It is time to let this informative and inspiring collection speak for itself.

Joan Chodorow

REFERENCES

Berrol, C. (2000). The spectrum of research options in dance/movement therapy. *American Journal of Dance Therapy, 22,* (1), 29–46.

Cruz, R. F., & Hervey, L. W. (2001). The American Dance Therapy Association research survey. *American Journal of Dance Therapy, 23,* (2), 89–118.

Hervey, L. W. (2000). *Artistic inquiry in dance/movement therapy: Creative research alternatives.* Springfield, IL: Charles C Thomas.

Jung, C. G. (1916/1958). The transcendent function. *Collected works*, Vol. 8, pp. 67–91. Princeton, NJ: Princeton University Press, 1975.

Whitehouse, M. (1958/1999). The Tao of the body. In P. Pallaro (Ed.), *Authentic Movement: Essays by Mary Starks Whitehouse, Janet Adler and Joan Chodorow*, (pp. 41–50). London: Jessica Kingsley.

ACKNOWLEDGMENTS

The editors gratefully acknowledge that indexing for this volume was provided through a grant from the Marian Chace Foundation of the American Dance Therapy Association.

CONTENTS

DANCE/MOVEMENT
THERAPISTS IN ACTION

Section 1

INTRODUCTION

Chapter 1

DIFFERENT CONCEPTUALIZATIONS OF RESEARCH: A READER'S GUIDE TO THIS TEXT

CYNTHIA F. BERROL AND ROBYN FLAUM CRUZ

Dance/movement therapists are immersed in the language of the body rather than focused solely on verbal communication. This concentration on dance/movement as a medium for mind/body healing—the distinguishing feature of the work that sets it apart from other types of therapy—is perhaps a factor in the ambivalent relationship practitioners have maintained with investigative research (see Feder & Feder, 1998; Cruz & Hervey, 2001; Higgens, 2001). The end result is reflected in the fact that the dance/movement therapy (DMT) literature is characterized by scant research publications in favor of theoretical contributions and practical descriptions. Interestingly, although the numbers of therapists and the populations they serve have increased over time, there has not been a commensurate increase in DMT publications that empirically support practice and theory.

Objective research has historically been perceived by dance/movement therapists as inherently incompatible with the process-oriented approach of DMT, tantamount to subjecting a personal, expressive experience to detached, microscopic scrutiny and analysis (Berrol, 2000). However, as the field has advanced over the last sixty years and spread to more than thirty-one countries around the globe, so too has awareness of the need for various kinds of scholarly research grown. Moreover, a number of American dance/movement therapists recently expressed a desire for improving their research skills and uniformly acknowledged the importance of research to the profession (Cruz & Hervey, 2001). Curiously, even though the literature of the human and behavioral sciences and various creative arts therapies features works devoted to research issues, DMT has failed to produce comparable writings, as evidenced by the dearth of published research studies. The literature focusing on the subject of research in the creative arts therapies consists primarily of the contributions of art and music therapists (Berrol, 2000).

A confluence of factors underscores the need for attention to research in DMT. The demands for accountability by health care insurance providers and other monitoring agencies have, in recent years, accelerated the necessity for assessment development and outcome research. Although the current thrust in many health care settings is for tangible evidence of treatment efficacy, many DMT practitioners lack the appropriate skills required for conducting investigative inquiry. A contributing issue has been the type of research methods to which DMT trainees have been exposed in the educational setting. Evidence from the American Dance Therapy Association research survey (Cruz & Hervey, 2001) indicated that dance/movement therapists have not been adequately prepared to explore the varied spectrum of inquiry options, no less to develop research projects in the clinical environment. Moreover, there is no single text that concentrates on the spectrum of artistic and scientific inquiry specifically directed to DMT. This volume is designed to fill that void.

With the field now ripe for a book about research directed to the dance/movement therapy community, we offer this edited text that spans and illuminates a breadth of investigative inquiry approaches and models. This volume highlights two basic research frameworks—quantitative (objective) and qualitative (interpretative)—including their underlying philosophic and theoretical tenets. Our goal has been to create a comprehensible, accessible book that is readable and engaging: one that contains accepted research protocols in conjunction with practical information written in "nontechnical" terms.

Many examples are incorporated throughout the text to clarify and amplify each of the various research options. We contend that there is no "one size fits all" model or any superiority of one paradigm over another, but rather, that the mindful matching of inquiry objectives and conditions with the appropriate methodological approaches creates valuable research. In this text, we aim to present a spectrum of research alternatives that can inform clinical practice, inspire the clinician, and guide further research inquiry.

OVERVIEW

This text is divided into four categorical sections, each containing related chapters. The first section, comprising this and another introductory chapter, provides a sequential guide to the contents of the volume and establishes a rationale for the relevance of research to the field of DMT. The second section explores "Traditional Methods and Research Considerations" and is primarily devoted to experimental designs and the alternatives within the quantitative research paradigm. The third segment, "Interpretative Methods and Research Considerations," addresses varying modes of qualitative approaches. A somewhat fluid form, interpretive designs continue to evolve to meet the changing conditions of research inquiry in the arts and behavioral sciences. The final section, "Creative

Alternatives and Options," comprises chapters that examine research alternatives and growing trends. These include a spectrum of research models and methods such as evaluation research, artistic inquiry, and mixing qualitative and quantitative methods in a single study.

Overview of Chapters

With respect to the organization of the text we should point out that within the different sections we set no specific criteria for the arrangement of chapters. Despite the careful thought given to their ordering, each chapter stands on its own merits and can be read independently of the others. However, when perusing a chapter, there are instances in which other chapters of the text are referenced, particularly when a specific aspect of the subject matter is fleshed-out more fully in the chapter cited than the one under perusal. Nevertheless, to obtain a comprehensive view of the multiple research options included and a satisfactory understanding of when and how they are applied, we recommend study of the entire volume.

Often, an individual's *interest* in a particular problem evokes questions that arouse her or his *curiosity*. The primary affect interest and its dynamic expression as curiosity (Stewart, 1987), in conjunction with the perceived importance of the emergent issue, are the catalysts that initially trigger the urge to probe further; that is, they are the initial stepping stones of research investigation. Illustrating the differing paths of research exploration, the chapters in this volume are designed to expose the therapist/researcher to tangible examples of the targeted method to help bridge the divide between research theory and practical application.

Chapter 2 (Cruz and Berrol) of Section 1 continues introducing this text by constructing a rationale to support why it is important for members of the DMT community—student, practitioner, or academician—to become actively involved in some form of research. We attempt to dispel the common mythology that frequently distances many dance/movement therapists from active engagement in investigative inquiry. Practical steps are introduced to prepare individuals for accessing and acquiring the resources necessary to undertake some form of research.

The overarching paradigms of deductive and inductive reasoning distinguish and shape the contrasting methods of quantitative and qualitative research, respectively. Chapters subsumed under Sections 2 and 3 illuminate the many facets of these two basic research frameworks, that is, introducing their respective theoretical and philosophic underpinnings and exploring the different research methods associated with each one.

Section 2 examines various approaches to quantitative research models. As a starting point, Chapter 3 (Berrol) concentrates on experimental design and its expanding options. In this chapter, Berrol traces the historical development of quantitative research through its transition into the more flexible research options of the latter part of the twentieth century. The chapter incorporates protocols and practical guidelines for designing studies for selected inquiry options and couples them with relevant examples.

Chapter 4 (Cruz and Koch) focuses on issues of validity and reliability in the use of movement observation scales. The authors offer practical suggestions and guidelines for using established observation instruments for DMT and for developing observation scales. Ways of using movement observation and explanation of the various types of validity and reliability issues that are important in the use of movement observation scales are discussed. The authors include information on an important reliability criterion, interrater agreement, amplifying and illustrating how this criterion may be calculated via the use of specific analytic methods.

Individual case study methods are presented in Chapter 5 (Chaiklin and Chaiklin). The authors examine what constitutes a "case," and when and how the case study is an effective method. They also discuss how case studies can be designed to present reliable and valid information that can be of value to others. By chronicling one therapist's work with an individual client, the authors illustrate how clinical practice can be transformed into valid case study research.

Single-subject design (SSD), featured in Chapter 6 (Goodill and Cruz), provides a logical follow-up to Chaiklin and Chaiklin's examination of individual case study methods by offering another pragmatic option for DMT. In addition to describing basic procedures for carrying out SSD research and its practical use to dance/movement therapists, the authors provide a comparison with individual case study research. A distinguishing aspect of the SSD approach is that it seeks to evaluate and demonstrate treatment effectiveness and likewise, to identify causal factors. Importantly, in SSD research the participant is compared to him- or herself during the different phases of the study, providing an efficient alternative to quantitative group designs where a control group is required for comparison.

The chapters of Section 3 contain an array of research approaches representing methods subsumed under the paradigm of qualitative research. The first, Chapter 7 (Green), offers readers a roadmap of the many subcategories of interpretive methods that have sprung up over the last twenty-five years. The author describes the subtleties of this new "territory" in ways that are often revelatory, and her focus on somatic sensitivity as a postpositivist research approach is concretized by her personal exploration of this form.

Chapter 8, "Qualitative Data Collection and Analysis" (Forinash), offers details of the entire procedure—from interviews and field observations to how collected data are analyzed. The author provides historical background regarding qualitative research and describes how the methods can be applied in different research settings. The process of qualitative research is thoughtfully illuminated by the narrative data of a project that explored the effects of DMT with older adults with mild Alzheimer's disease.

Chapter 9 (Hanna) on anthropological methods in DMT research places issues relating to DMT within a sociocultural context. The author addresses how an anthropological approach can assist dance/movement therapists in discovering ways of working with and conducting studies with different groups in accordance with their respective cultural beliefs and practices.

The final section of the book begins with Chapter 10 (Cruz) on evaluation research. Evaluation offers a pragmatic approach that dance/movement therapists can use to support and extend the treatment programs they offer. Cruz demonstrates how evaluation research assists in determining the merits of a program and in shaping policy. The example of a program evaluation project funded by the Marian Chace Foundation of the American Dance Therapy Association is offered to illustrate the process and inspire dance/movement therapists to undertake this type of research.

Chapter 11 (Hervey) addresses artistic inquiry in DMT and should be of particular interest to dance/movement therapists. Currently gaining recognition in the creative arts therapies, this method embodies a process-oriented mode for exploring, developing, and analyzing research issues directly through an art form. In addition to explicating the concepts and methods of artistic inquiry, Hervey illustrates the method by recounting the actual experiences of a gradate student as she progressed through the stages of developing, implementing, and analyzing her artistic inquiry research project.

Chapter 12 (Berrol) describes how quantitative and qualitative methods can be used in varying combinations in a single DMT research project. Mixing methods has been portrayed as an approach that conceivably extends the dimensions and depth of a study. Berrol provides background on this emergent form and describes how mixed methods research and/or paradigms can be incorporated into an investigative inquiry or during different phases of its gestation. A selected group of research studies are presented to illustrate how mixed methods can be integrated into an investigative inquiry.

Although the final chapter focuses on combining methods within a single project, the text as a whole scrutinizes, explains, and offers examples of each of the respective methods. Aptly, Politsky (1995) applied a psychological lens to the differing research paradigms, superimposing on them an intrapsychic typology reflective of Jung's ego functions (thinking, sensing, feeling, and intuiting). She posited that quantitative research represents the ego functions of thinking and sensing while the typology of interpretive research mirrors the ego functions of feeling and intuition. Extending this model metaphorically, we propose that the two research paradigms embody all four ego functions; that together they create a balance in which one paradigm informs and completes the other. Such a union has the potential to build a body of knowledge that at once presents concrete outcome data and yet captures the substance and meaning of the therapeutic process (Berrol, 2000). This core premise reflects the basic tenets of the text: that is, a multifaceted view of the possibilities of research inquiry—one that extends far beyond the commonly held perceptions of what it is and how it is conducted.

It is our opinion that the nature of this material is essential to students preparing thesis research in DMT graduate programs. Further, we believe that these chapters hold a wealth of information and examples that will be of particular use and interest to clinicians. Many chapters were conceived and written with practitioners in mind, for example, one featuring the use of movement observation scales for DMT research and clinical practice, and one on using research results to inform clinical practice. We trust that this volume will afford dance/movement therapists the tools to conduct research related to both clinical practice and academic inquiry. However, our personal hope is that it kindles excitement and a sense of empowerment about research in all of our DMT colleagues, and inspires a new generation of dance/movement therapist/researchers.

REFERENCES

Berrol, C. F. (2000). The spectrum of research options in dance/movement therapy. *American Journal of Dance Therapy, 22*(1), 29–46.

Cruz, R. F., & Hervey, L. W. (2001). The American Dance Therapy Association research survey. *American Journal of Dance Therapy,* 23(2), 89–118.

Feder, B., & Feder, E. (1998). *The art and science of evaluation in the arts therapies.* Springfield, IL: Charles C Thomas.

Higgens, L. (2001). On the value of conducting dance/movement therapy research. *The Arts in Psychotherapy, 28*(3), 191–195.

Politsky, R. H. (1995). Toward a typology of research in the creative arts therapies. *The Arts in Psychotherapy, 22*(4), 307–314.

Stewart, L. H. (1987). A brief report: Affect and archetype. *Journal of Analytical Psychology, 32,* 35–46.

Chapter 2

WHAT DOES RESEARCH HAVE TO DO WITH IT?

ROBYN FLAUM CRUZ AND CYNTHIA F. BERROL

Like other clinicians, dance/movement therapists spend many hours in training, learning to deliver good clinical care to the individuals they treat. In addition, most also spend long hours in the first years of practice seeking supervision to improve their clinical skills. Some dance/movement therapists participate in ongoing supervision after the required hours for registry with the American Dance Therapy Association (ADTA) have been completed; they attend conferences, postgraduate education programs, and read professional journals such as the *American Journal of Dance Therapy*. So how does research fit into this ongoing search for clinical excellence? Is research really useful or necessary to clinical practice, or does it have a different purpose?

We will examine these questions, but as this chapter helps introduce an entire volume devoted to describing different methods of research, we want to open with a brief definition of research. Williams and Irving succinctly described research as "simply a critical systematic process of inquiry: its aim is to move from opinion to knowledge" (Williams & Irving, 1999, p. 368). This general definition is useful for our purposes because, as will be demonstrated in other chapters, there is no one type of science, conceptual framework, or research method that is recommended over any other; in this volume it is our intent to present the pluralism of approaches to research that are available. We do agree with Williams and Irving that "what is important [regardless of research approach] is that research findings are valid and reliable" (p. 368), meaning that research propositions should be corroborated in ways congruent with other knowledge and dependable regardless of approach used. We, and the authors represented in this volume, present more in-depth definitions of research and the different approaches that can be used. However, the brief definition above suffices for the purpose of discussing the interface of research and practice.

THE INTERFACE OF RESEARCH AND PRACTICE

Historically, clinicians in a range of different disciplines have had uneasy relationships with research and understanding how to use research to

11

inform practice. Some clinicians report that published research results seem unrelated to clinical practice. They may fail to recognize that information about group behavior and characteristics may be readily transformed into knowledge that can be applied to the individual clients they see. In fact, many therapists fail to use research results to inform their clinical practice, a phenomenon that is not unique to a particular discipline, and one that has been discussed in psychology, marriage and family therapy, counseling and guidance, and other psychotherapy professions including arts therapies (Goldfried & Wolfe, 1996; Johnson, Sandberg, & Miller, 1999; Williams & Irving, 1999; Polkinghorne, 1999; Cruz & Hervey, 2001).

In psychology, doctoral training programs have used a scientist/practitioner model in which students are required to actively participate in and produce research whether they plan to practice primarily as clinicians or researchers. While it was hoped that this would produce clinicians who use research results to inform their practice, data indicate that this has not had the desired effect (Goldfried & Wolfe, 1996).

In dance/movement therapy (DMT), similar issues about how to apply research results to treatment, as well as other factors, contribute to how dance/movement therapists relate or do not relate to research. Results of the ADTA Research Survey (Cruz & Hervey, 2001) indicated that dance/movement therapists often have more questions than answers about research. The dance therapists who were surveyed seemed to feel that research was important to the profession rather than to their practices.

Many clinicians report that they fail to see the relevance of published research results to clinical practice. Therapists' indifference to research has been discussed over the last fifty years, and many perspectives and suggestions to deal with this indifference have been presented. But why is there concern about therapists' lack of attention to research? The answer lies in the fact that psychotherapy practice relies to a great extent on the individual practitioner's skills in assessing, interpreting, and intervening with accuracy so that the client is guided in a process of inter- and intrapersonal growth. Therapists carefully watch and listen, collecting information from clients and forming hypotheses or educated guesses involving predictions about what issues, directions, and interventions might move the client forward toward health. The therapist then tests these hypotheses by actually making interventions and noting the client's response or lack of response. In a sense, clinical practice is similar to an ongoing experiment, as the therapist is continually collecting and analyzing data. Chaiklin and Chaiklin (Chapter 5 of this volume) support in some detail a practical case for viewing clinical practitioners as already involved in the process of doing research. They illustrate how a dance/movement therapist's clinical work with a client can be transformed into case study research.

The reason we emphasize the importance of incorporating research into clinical practice is that it helps clinicians generate better working hypotheses by expanding their resources for thinking about cases and advancing their clinical skills. Consider the complexity of the task of treatment and note that clinicians must not only consider individual development, history, personality, and symptoms but must also integrate other equally complicated factors such as culture, race, family structure, ethics, and treatment philosophy into their work. What makes this highly complex process both possible and effective, is the efforts of the therapist to generate working hypotheses that are based on knowledge and comparative data. When this happens, work with each client in each session is both supported and enhanced. From this viewpoint, the very process of treatment can be considered an aspect of or preparation for research.

How Does Research Affect Practice?

While each therapist conceivably builds a base of knowledge through practice, imagine how inefficient it would be for each therapist to work only from his or her own experiences. The therapist who works only from the knowledge base of personal experience becomes locked within the parameters of his or her somewhat limited world view. Psychotherapists, including dance/movement therapists, are introduced to many theoretical approaches, compilations of facts, and information about human psychological processes during their education. Just as this information forms a base for beginning practice, research forms a base for the further development of theoretical and factual knowledge.

We want to examine the term *knowledge* briefly because it plays an important role in our arguments for using research to inform clinical practice. Epistemology refers to the ideas people hold about what counts as knowledge—the information that they judge as constituting evidence for a claim, and what warrants that evidence. Everyone has personal epistemologies that have been influenced by their histories including, but not limited to, their formal education. The individual nature of epistemologies means that not everyone will agree on what counts as evidence for a claim or what constitutes knowledge. As in many other aspects of life, diversity in epistemologies is healthy. What is important for the dance/movement therapist engaging in clinical practice and research, is an understanding of his or her criteria for what constitutes knowledge and an awareness of how this understanding develops or changes as new information is learned. We hope that the chapters in this volume assist dance/movement therapists in this process of defining and extending knowledge.

With respect to another important term, *theories*, we want to point out that useful theories are those that state expectations or relationships between ideas that can be explored. Exploration consists of looking not only for data that support the theorized relationship or expectation, but even more importantly, looking for data that do not fit the proposed model or mold. The true usefulness of research lies in posing a question, searching among the possible answers, and attempting to rule out some of them to narrow the field of answers. As the reader may have guessed from this description, research is a process of continually refining knowledge and understanding by seeking information that does and *does not* confirm the researchers' hypotheses or the theories they entertain. In fact, we argue that looking for unusual cases or instances that do not fit the therapist's or researcher's hypotheses is a most efficient approach to inquiry. The process of refining knowledge and theory was referred to in the definition of research by Williams and Irving (1999) at the beginning of this chapter, because it describes the movement from opinion to knowledge that is the goal of research. Higgens (2001) went further by identifying the purpose of scholarly research in dance/movement therapy specifically, as creating *new* knowledge.

One of the primary concerns expressed regarding therapists' indifference to research is that when practitioners rely on personal opinion, nonaxiomatic truths, and loosely construed and personalized theories, practice is not refined or improved (Williams & Irving, 1999). We alluded to this when we mentioned the limitations of a therapist who only works from a personal knowledge base rather than the knowledge base of the field. Practitioners are vulnerable to pitfalls that can undermine their work when they substitute opinion or a system of beliefs for knowledge, because beliefs cannot be disproved and disproving, as we mentioned, is a vital element for research and accumulating knowledge. The substitution of opinion for knowledge is a tempting trap, as it can masquerade, undetected, as one's truth. Williams and Irving created a classification of the inherent pitfalls when practitioners are indifferent to research: (a) epistemology—reliance on personal knowledge that may be shared with no one thus making it difficult to judge its validity; (b) preciousness—reliance on nonaxiomatic truths, beliefs, or emotionally held ideas to the exclusion of information to the contrary; (c) lack of theoretical rigor—looseness with which constructs are construed rather than using them within a defined theoretical framework; (d) non-Popperian logic—a tendency to work within a theory and defend it regardless of other evidence; and (e) personalization of theory—seeing evaluation or evaluative thinking about practice and theories as criticism.

As commented upon earlier, clinicians frequently complain that research seems unrelated to their practices. Yet, research and clinical practice are actually linked by their mutual dependence on a systematic body of knowledge. So for example, any failure of research impedes the ability of the professional to function, and limitations in clinical practice fail to provide the necessary direction to researchers (Striker, 1992). This interface and interaction between practitioners and researchers is of such importance that many studies have focused on attempting to understand how and why it is underutilized. In one study, clinicians complained that published research lacked relevance to their practices, but when the researchers reviewed the contemporary research in that field to support the clinicians' complaint, they found that in fact there had been efforts made in most articles to report *practical implications* of findings in concluding remarks (Nicholas & Gilbert, 1980). In another study, results indicated that clinicians' attitudes toward research were positively influenced by contact with a significant mentor during training (Anderson, 1999). On the other hand, a documented view by practitioners contends that research is somehow antithetical to the values or the artistic nature of psychotherapy (Shipton, 1996; Forrester, 1997). The relationship of research to clinical practitioners appears to be complex, but is nonetheless significant as it impacts the development and growth of clinically oriented professions such as dance/movement therapy.

Research and DMT Practitioners

Research became an important component of education, psychology, and medicine—shaping practices and principles—over the last 100 years. Fueled by developments in the philosophy of science, statistical, and other techniques in the first part of the twentieth century (Anastasi, 1988), inquiry in the social sciences is ever increasing. Many models and approaches to research have gained acceptance (Bogdan & Biklen, 1992), and advances in knowledge have been applied across the mental health professions.

When DMT developed in the 1940s as a formal practice (Bartenieff, 1972–1973), the early DMT literature was made up of theoretical formulations and practice descriptions (see, for example, Chace, 1953). Research-oriented publications were added to the literature as the new profession evolved, and the first issue of the *American Journal of Dance Therapy* was published in 1977 (Stark, 2002). While studies using group designs have been published over the years, in 1996 the case study was noted to be the most popular DMT research method (Ritter & Low, 1996). DMT research is featured in a range of journals, but it can be argued that the volume of DMT research is not in step with the demands of ethical practice and health care policy. As an example, between 1998 and 2000, only three inquiry-based articles were published in the *American Journal of Dance Therapy*. We briefly discussed results of the survey of attitudes of dance/movement therapists toward research (Cruz & Hervey, 2001) earlier. An important part of the results of this survey pointed to the necessary focus of DMT training on preparation for clinical practice rather than on research or the combination of the two, as a factor likely limiting dance/movement therapists' relationships to research.

Dance/movement therapists are trained in two-year master's degree programs in which preparation for clinical practice is the main focus of the curriculum. After graduation, most dance/movement therapists work in clinical practice settings where the immediacy of the therapeutic moment and demands of the setting can take precedence over all other activities. These factors, among others, presumably contribute to limiting how dance/movement therapists relate to research. While a course in research is required for dance/movement therapy training programs, in most instances the goal is to prepare students to complete thesis research and these courses do not give individuals enough understanding of research to support its use in professional dance/movement therapy practice. Some evidence from the ADTA research survey (Cruz & Hervey, 2001) supports this assertion, including the fact that most survey respondents did not feel their dance/movement therapy training prepared them for undertaking research or professional writing. In addition, many of the dance/movement therapists surveyed were uncertain of the value of research to their own practices, and few had exposure to the full range of research methods in their educations. While it is unrealistic to expect two-year programs to educate practitioner/scientists, graduate-level teachers and mentors are a vitally important resource to positively influence dance/movement therapy students with regard to research. In addition, continuing education, from conference attendance to pursuing higher degrees, can have a positive impact on professional dance/movement therapists' views of and relationships to research.

The idea for this book grew out of the same initiative as the ADTA research survey (Cruz & Hervey, 2001) in which the ADTA Research Committee members sought to better understand how dance/movement therapists relate or do not relate to research. Results of the study gave a further spark to our idea as many respondents reported that they had an interest in research but did not feel that they had sufficient understanding of or exposure to research methods to pursue their research ideas. In addition, some respondents who had returned to school for advanced degrees remarked on the greater acceptance of a wider range of methods for research than they had known about previously, and reported feeling both empowered and more excited about research with this new knowledge.

A related factor fomenting the genesis of this volume was the striking realization that a number of publications involving the creative arts therapies were starting to probe the nature of research inquiry, rather than concentrating exclusively on reporting research outcomes, as customary. Focusing on the creative arts, these articles and books were predominantly the work of art and music therapists, and examined underlying philosophical, theoretical, and methodological tenets as well as the diverse research options open to the creative arts therapies. Interestingly, not a single manuscript was directed specifically to DMT, nor was there one authored by a dance/movement therapist (Berrol, 2000).

Thus, the purpose of this volume is both to expose dance/movement therapists to methodology presented in somewhat discrete chapters of possible research methods for the discipline, and excite readers about the many possibilities for inquiry in DMT. The link we described earlier between research and practice is not simply a fanciful notion; it is a reality that we believe all dance/movement therapists experience everyday. We ask the reader to take a moment and think about the last DMT session that he or she conducted. What types of issues arose? What questions were posed in the dance/movement therapist's mind after the clients left the session? Were these new questions or questions that have risen before? This process of identifying questions about DMT work is the core of research inquiry.

All research begins simply by generating questions and desiring answers. Research is the process of searching for answers to questions by developing a systematic approach to inquiry or exploration. Meekums (1996, p. 130) wrote that research is an "act of creation" or a creative process that possesses all the elements of excitement and fulfillment that are associated with other creative processes. Dibbel-Hope (2000) described the compelling journey she made in pursuit of her doctoral research from her initial identification of the research question through completion of the project. From her description, it is easy to identify the creative fulfillment she gained during the process. This has certainly been one of the greatest motivators for our own individual endeavors with research. Examining the validity of Davis' Movement Psychodiagnostic Inventory (Cruz, 1995) was the culmination of more than fifteen years of fascination with involuntary movement disorders and their potential as diagnostic indicators. Thousands of hours spent exploring data, literature, and collaborating with colleagues and mentors seemed to fly by, and it is hard to describe how something so all-consuming can produce such a sense of *aliveness* and total stimulation. The excitement of exploration and discovery and the hours of puzzling through problems can be some of the most stimulating and professionally fulfilling experiences—and we intend this volume to similarly stimulate and excite readers about participating in research. The professional growth that dance/movement therapists experience through research activities is of benefit to the entire profession. We want to begin our encouragement to dance/movement therapists by suggesting a few simple ways of introducing research into clinical practice.

INCLUDING RESEARCH IN PRACTICE AND BECOMING A THERAPIST/RESEARCHER

Because work with clients frequently presents questions to the therapist, these questions offer one way to begin incorporating research into one's practice. One's questions can begin to define a particular area of interest and generate other questions. Colleagues and supervisors are a useful first resource for investigating questions as they often can recommend articles or books (note that references in a single suggested article will lead to related literature in that subject area). Searching for information on a topic is actually a form of inquiry, so at this early juncture the therapist becomes a researcher. Other resources available to the therapist/researcher range from research courses at local community colleges to Internet resources, such as full text journals online that can be accessed with a home computer. Likewise, the ADTA electronic mail list promotes the sharing of information, ideas and resources that are helpful to the germination of research projects.

Journal clubs in which colleagues meet regularly to read and discuss articles are particularly helpful for increasing understanding of published research results and how to apply these to practice, because members collaborate and share information with each other. This is also a good way to develop more comfort with reading certain types of research that may use terminology (for example, statistical language) that is not very familiar. Using the collective and interactive resources of a group can make decoding and learning more productive and fun than simply studying alone. The inclusion of therapists from other disciplines can also enhance a journal club by bringing different perspectives together. While it is good to look for research articles in dance therapy, seminal information outside the field is applicable to dance/movement therapy and should not be overlooked, and the creative synthesis of the process becomes more exciting with the breadth of information found.

Research truly is a creative and interactive pursuit, and beginning simply with colleagues and questions soon moves to identifying and refining a research query worthy of in-depth development. We hope this text stimulates interest in exploring questions and assists dance/movement therapists in discovering answers through the various facets and phases of the research inquiry process. Truly, individual therapists, the clients they treat, and the profession will all benefit from research exploration.

REFERENCES

Anastasi, A. (1988). *Psychological testing*. (6th ed.) New York: Macmillan.

Anderson, S. E. (1999). Critical incidents in the development of research attitudes among counseling psychology graduate students. *Dissertation Abstracts International Section A: Humanities and Social Sciences. 60* (2-A), 03331.

Bartenieff, I. (1972-1973). Dance therapy: A new profession or a rediscovery of an ancient role of the dance? *Dance Scope, 7* (Fall–Winter, 1972–1973), 6–18.

Berrol, C., F. (2000). The spectrum of research options in dance/movement therapy. *American Journal of Dance Therapy, 22*(1), 29–46.

Bogdan, R. C., & Biklen, S. K. (1992). *Qualitative research for education*. (2nd ed.) Boston: Allyn and Bacon.

Chace, M. (1953). Dance as an adjunctive therapy with hospitalized mental patients. *Bulletin of the Menninger Clinic, 17,* 219–225.

Cruz, R. F. (1995). An empirical investigation of the Movement Psychodiagnostic Inventory. (Doctoral dissertation, The University of Arizona). *Dissertation Abstracts International, (2B), (UMI No.AAM962042257)*.

Cruz, R. F., & Hervey, L. W. (2001). The American Dance Therapy Association research survey. *American Journal of Dance Therapy, 23*(2), 89–118.

Dibbel-Hope, S. (2000). From DTR to PhD: The personal story of my dissertation, *Moving Toward Health. American Journal of Dance Therapy, 22*(1), 61–77.

Forrester, D. (1997). Letter to the editor. *Counseling, 8*, 224.

Goldfried, M. R., & Wolfe, B. E. (1996). Psychotherapy practice and research: Repairing a strained alliance. *American Psychologist, 51*, 1007–1016.

Higgens, L. (2001). On the value of conducting dance/movement therapy research. *The Arts in Psychotherapy, 28*, 191–195.

Johnson, L., Sandberg, J., & Miller, R. (1999). Research practices of marriage and family therapists. *The American Journal of Family Therapy, 27*, 239–249.

Meekums, B. (1996). Research as an act of creation. In H. Payne (Ed.), *Handbook of inquiry in arts therapies,* (pp. 130–137). London: Jessica Kingsley.

Nicholas, M. J., & Gilbert, J. P. (1980). Research in music therapy: A survey of music therapists' attitudes and knowledge. *Journal of Music Therapy, 17*, 207–213.

Polkinghorne, D. (1999). Traditional research and psychotherapy practice. *Journal of Clinical Psychology, 55*, 1429–1440.

Ritter, M., & Low, K. G. (1996). The effectiveness of dance/movement therapy. *The Arts in Psychotherapy, 23*(3), 249–260.

Shipton, G. (1996). Working with resistance to research. In S. Palmer, S. Dainow, & P. Milner (Eds.), *Counseling: The BAC counseling reader* (pp. 539–545). London: Sage.

Stark, A. (2002). The American Journal of Dance Therapy: Its history and evolution. *American Journal of Dance Therapy, 24* (2), 73–95.

Striker, G. (1992). The relationship of research to clinical practice. *American Psychologist, 47*, 543–549.

Williams, D. I., & Irving J. A. (1999). Symposium: Why are therapists indifferent to research? *British Journal of Guidance & Counseling, 27*, 367–376.

Section 2

TRADITIONAL METHODS

AND RESEARCH CONSIDERATIONS

Chapter 3

THE EXPANDING OPTIONS OF
EXPERIMENTAL RESEARCH DESIGN IN
DANCE/MOVEMENT THERAPY

CYNTHIA F. BERROL

Whether as children or adults, we are involved in various sorts of investigative inquiry: we observe, analyze, and interpret our world on some level. It's certainly true for the dance/movement therapist in clinical practice. A major distinction between day-to-day clinical and scientific problem solving is that the latter extends beyond the particular interests or needs of an individual or therapist to embrace an entire discipline.

Research means careful critical inquiry and examination for the purpose of discovery and interpretation of new knowledge. It exists in various forms, from the deductive reasoning paradigm undergirding quantitative and quasi-experimental research to inductive models using interpretive, qualitative approaches. A key concern in any research inquiry is that the goals and objectives of a study correspond with the selected methods—that an appropriate match has been made. Thus the research model hinges on the purpose of the study and types of questions posed and not vice versa (Guralnik, 1992; Tashakkori & Teddlie, 1998; Cresswell, 1994).

Prior to the emergence and proliferation of the social sciences, research concentrated exclusively on observable elements of the physical world and the laws of nature. Studies were grounded in "analytic empiricism," namely, observation and analysis under a carefully formulated set of controlled conditions. However, the accelerated growth of the human sciences in the twentieth century not only expanded the parameters of quantitative options but, likewise, spawned the development of well-structured qualitative research methods which are presented in other chapters in this volume (Tashakkori & Teddlie, 1998; Cresswell, 1994; Borg, Gall, & Gall, 1993).

This chapter begins with a focus on the scientific approaches of experimental research and its more contemporary offshoot, quasi-experimental design, now commonly used in the behavioral sciences and the arts. One caution: the content included here is not intended to cover the vast scope of the scientific model; the contents are limited to key features important for basic insights into and understanding of the underpinnings of this paradigm, and likewise, as a stepping stone into research procedures.

The Scientific (Positivistic) Model

In recent years, various media, professional journals, and newsletters have devoted much attention to the ramifications of the rapidly changing health care system and the need for accountability through research. Importantly, not only have these external sources spawned pressure regarding the call for research in dance/movement therapy (DMT) and the other creative arts therapies, internal growth and development within the respective modalities have directed attention to research issues. McNiff (1987) contends that "every profession has needs for quantification and operational statistics" (p. 286). Feder and Feder (1998) opine that while the arts represent the essence of humanity, science helps determine appropriate treatment for particular individuals and groups, and even more elemental, verifies whether the treatment works.

Scientific or positivistic research (as it is also known) embraces measurable, observable phenomena related to the human experience and the natural world. It is based on the assumption that natural phenomena behave in orderly, predictable ways and that the business of science is to gather facts to explain these laws of nature. The essence of quantitative research is to generate research derived, initially, from questions that are then formulated into hypotheses (Kerlinger, 1973; Simon, 1969; Chatfield, 1999; Cook & Campbell, 1979).

A benchmark of the positivistic paradigm is a mode of reasoning whose lineage dates back to the ancient world in which Aristotelian logic was the ideal model. This is a paradigm founded on deductive reasoning, a type of abstract thinking that hypothesizes—that is, predicts or explains the specific consequences of a set of causal relationships—and proceeds to verify them by adhering to a systematic set of conditions. In other words, this type of logic sets out to confirm (or refute) theoretically derived predictions regarding selected phenomena (Kerlinger, 1973). Deductive analysis begins with a problem or theoretical question from which an hypothesis is formulated. Armed with documentation from the literature, knowledge, experience, and imagination, the researcher deduces likely sequelae of the generated hypothesis.

Objectivity and critical thinking are the hallmarks of the positivistic model. Rooted in scientific methods, it is frequently concerned with experimental designs and measurable outcomes. The researcher wants to discover facts upon which to advance theories that minimize human biases, and to develop and test hypotheses using objective methods (Borg & Gall, 1979; Politsky, 1995). A set of tightly structured research protocols is followed to test the validity of specific theoretical constructs. As a paradigm designed to shape and augment the extant body of knowledge, these procedures strive to establish the truthfulness of a hypothetical proposition, that is, its credibility and integrity or validity (Aldridge & Aldridge, 1996). Validity and accuracy of outcomes are further verified through replication studies conducted to rule out rival causal theories (Politsky, 1995; Kerlinger, 1973; Campbell & Stanley, 1966). The process is devised to validate predictions and generalize outcomes. In this way, as theories are tested, verified, and amplified, they shape and augment the existing body of knowledge. Table 3-I encapsulates the basic characteristics of quantitative research generally associated with this paradigm.

Table 3-I   BASIC CHARACTERISTICS OF QUANTITATIVE RESEARCH

Categories	Quantitative Research : Experimental and Quasi-experimental Designs
Goals of researcher	Facts, truths, and explanations related to natural and behavioral sciences
Paradigm	Deductive reasoning based on established theoretical constructs
Type of data collected	Typically quantifiable, outcome oriented, verifiable, reliable
Type of data analysis	Statistical analyses: frequencies, correlations, inferential statistics—often involves causal relationships; comparisons of two or more groups on selected variables
Characteristics of researcher	Objective researcher, removed from data; works from without; non-interactive observer
Characteristics of research	Objective, value free, rational, accurate, valid, reliable, factual
Attributes of research models	Deductive paradigm—hypothesis testing; reductionist (tries to rule out or eliminate alternative causal theories); interpretive, based on data finding; inferential
Goals of research	Generalizability with adequate replication studies; predictions and inferences; amplification and /or formulations of theory

Note: Ideas were derived from Cook and Reichardt (1979, p. 10); and Politsky (1995, pp. 308–809).

Quasi-experimental Research

Characterized as a theory-driven, deductive approach, there is currently more flexibility vis-à-vis research protocols than in previous eras. Scientists of early periods explored the laws of nature, conducting their experiments in laboratory settings where the phenomena under observation could be manipulated and tested under tightly controlled conditions. Borg, Gall, and Gall (1993) rightly contend that the behavioral sciences—the study of human organisms—are inherently more complex than the physical sciences or the study of objects and things. Multiple theories have evolved to explicate a vast range of behaviors on a continuum stretching from infancy to old age with respect to all the domains of human function. The difficulty lies in teasing out and controlling for the different internal and external conditions that can impact individual and group behavior and performance. Linear causal relationships, held to be facts or truths in the physical science realm, do not as readily translate to the human sciences. Simply, the intricate interweaving web of factors creates problems in juggling all the tenable possibilities. Behavioral studies conducted in the real world—outside the realm of the neatly configured laboratory setting—are subject to the complexities of existential dynamics, a fact that has had a tangible impact on empirical research.

Recognition of these realities paved the way for quasi-experimental research, a more practical approach for the arts and human sciences. Thus the preponderance of behavioral studies fall into the category of quasi-experimental research. This means that most studies can only approximate the conditions of pure experimental designs in that for one or more reasons they fail to meet the necessary criteria. Since the scientific model is predicated on rigorously configured and controlled empirical evidence (Kerlinger, 1973), any relevant variables beyond the control of the researcher necessitate methodological compromises. In quasi-experimental research, the investigator not only needs to be aware of, but also to work within the constraints of this modified form (Isaac & Michael, 1981; see also Chapter 12 in this volume). Although there is no one final word on any inquiry, the researcher must be mindful of the procedural limitations of a study and candid in disclosing its weaknesses and consequent implications.

Regardless of the model implemented, the standards linked to a particular approach are observed. This chapter will focus on experimental research, embracing its more contemporary companion, quasi-experimental research design; related validity and reliability issues will likewise be reviewed. In this chapter, the generic term *experimental design* will be applied to both experimental and quasi-experimental inquiries. Two alternative modes within the domain of scientific research methods—descriptive and historical research—will be briefly addressed as well.

THE RESEARCH PROCESS

Basic Guidelines for Developing a Research Proposal and Doing Research

First and foremost the researcher identifies issues of personal interest to explore: an idea that both inspires questions and requires in-depth investigation. Ideas frequently emerge from one's experiences in the field coupled with knowledge of the literature. Importantly, there should be a compelling reason for posing and researching the question, that is, a reason that transcends the individual and impacts the profession as a whole.

After the research question has been determined, the process truly gets underway. The researcher: 1) establishes a valid rationale; 2) clearly formulates and states the research question; 3) carefully reviews the literature for information pertinent to the study; 4) formulates operational definitions for the variables on which the study is based; 5) confronts issues of validity and reliability; 6) fleshes-out selected methods and procedures; 7) conducts statistical analyses of the data and reports results; 8) discusses and interprets results, and makes inferences; 9) draws conclusions and suggests directions for future research. These fundamental elements will be more fully delineated below.

1. The Rationale

One of the first steps of research is to develop a framework for the study. Typically, this means background information about the topic that helps justify why the inquiry is needed and its potential significance to the field. Similarly, related research is cited to build a solid case to support the rationale. Often a project is undertaken to replicate previous research, as a single study does not provide "necessary and sufficient evidence" (Cook & Campbell, 1979, p. 12) to confirm its findings; the undergirding motive is to rule out or eliminate possible competing theories that might weaken or refute its theoretical constructs. Problems that place single studies into question may range from methodological flaws and limitations to questions left unanswered. Or, a researcher may seek to clarify or amplify important aspects of prior inquiries. These sorts of reasons form the constituents of the "Statement of the Problem" and "Statement of Purpose," and both are intrinsic to the preparatory phase of the process.

Another essential element of this preliminary phase is a crystallization of assumptions and/or theories. Neuman & Benz (1998) caution researchers that assumptions should be based on credible theory. Dance/movement therapists have only to reflect on common clinical practices and the spectrum of well established psychosocial theories in which they are rooted— Jungian, Freudian, Adlerian, Piagetian, and the models spawned from them. All, in fact, are predicated upon a collection of assumptions based on observations and experiences associated with various domains of human development and function. However, for a theory to be accepted as fact, it must undergo rigorous and repeated testing under controlled conditions.

2. The Hypothesis

In experimental inquiry, research questions are reframed into hypotheses, a way of stating the relationship between variables so that they can be tested (Walizer & Wienir, 1978). Essentially these are logically evolved predictions about relationships between the factors being tested under controlled conditions (see hypothesis stating example below). This mode of abstract reasoning conjectures that "if" something (a causal factor, i.e., the independent

variable) is acted upon in a particular way, "then" a predicted type of consequence will occur in its counterpart (i.e., the dependent variable) that is
both observable and measurable (Kerlinger, 1973; Campbell & Stanley, 1966;
Cook & Reichardt, 1979; Neuman & Benz, 1998; Cresswell, 1994).

Research hypotheses can be stated in two ways, either as nondirectional
or directional. The first predicts that *some* difference will be discerned
between or among the related variables, and the second predicts that a *specified* difference will be observed, for example, that one group will perform
better or worse than another group studied.

The example that follows illustrates how an hypothesis ties together the
way in which an *independent* variable explains or predicts the outcome of the
dependent variable in a causal relationship—that is, by way of a logical,
abstract ("if—then") prediction. The example begins with the research
question followed by the two types of hypotheses.

1) **Research Question:**
   Does DMT help reduce anxiety in those individuals who have high levels of anxiety?

2) **Nondirectional Research Hypothesis:**
   If one group of individuals identified with high levels of anxiety is
   exposed to DMT and a comparable group is exposed to creative dance
   activities, *differences* in level of anxiety will be discerned between the
   two groups.

3) **Directional Research Hypothesis:**
   If one group of individuals identified with high levels of anxiety is
   exposed to DMT and a comparable group is exposed to creative dance
   activities, the group receiving the DMT will reveal a *greater reduction* in
   anxiety on selected anxiety measures than the group receiving creative
   dance activities.

In this example, the *independent variable* embraces two possible interventions: DMT or creative dance activities. The *dependent variable* is anxiety, and
if additional anxiety measures were to be used, they would all constitute
dependent variables. It's important to understand that independent and
dependent variables constitute the infrastructures of theoretical constructs.
In causal relationship research, one begins with an effect and attempts to
verify its cause (i.e., the independent variable) that is hypothesized to trigger the observable effect (i.e. change in the dependent variable). So in the
sample hypotheses above, the selected anxiety tests would be the criteria
employed to determine the effect of the intervention. Statistical tests are
conducted to evaluate the research hypothesis against a statistical prediction of no change—commonly referred to as the "null hypothesis."[1]

---

[1]An example of how a null hypothesis might be stated is: If a group of individuals identified with high
levels of anxiety is exposed to dance movement therapy and a comparable group is exposed to creative dance activities, there will be no differences revealed between the two on a measure of anxiety.

If the predicted difference between groups (known as the experimental effect) is detected by the statistical test of the data (meaning that we are able to reject the null hypothesis), we state that the result is statistically significant. While an explication of statistics is beyond the scope of this chapter, it is important to understand that the researcher sets the level of probability for assessing what is acceptable as statistical significance and further, that statistical significance implies that the results obtained from the statistical tests are not likely to be random occurrences (Borg, Gall, & Gall, 1993; Neuman & Benz, 1998). Nevertheless, it is necessary to also understand that even a high level of confidence in the statistical outcome does not prove an hypothesis, it merely supports it. Cook and Campbell (1979) maintain that scientific truths are never proven with logical certainty. Replication studies are needed to rule out competing explanations, a process used to strengthen external validity— meaning to augment the integrity of generalizations and inferences. Statistically significant findings do not establish a cause/effect relationship per se; rather, they simply establish levels of probability associated with the data at hand (see Chapter 6 in this text for more discussion of causality).

3. Review of Literature

The cornerstone of all research, the literature review implies a thorough exploration and evaluation of extant studies and recognized theoretical constructs directly related to the research topic. The process helps establish the rationale for the study and may lead to unexplored possibilities that help generate new ideas. In other words, it lays the groundwork that will shape and support the research procedures and methods, and guide its direction. The information gleaned serves to expand one's knowledge base, reveal what's already been done, and to expose strengths and weaknesses of previous works. Importantly, the confluence of propositions discovered in the literature helps construct a viable theoretical framework for the germinal stage of the process (Chatfield, 1999; Reis & Judd, 2000).

A good illustration of a well-conceived review of literature can be found in an article based on the observations of an art therapist working in a hospital with individuals with anorexia nervosa. Rehavia-Hanauer (2003) identified and illuminated conflictual issues associated with this disorder. Her research is well documented by a review of literature that spans a spectrum of theoretical models dealing with the genesis of anorexia. The theories reviewed incorporated a range of models: developmental, psychoanalytic, psychodynamic, object relations, sociocultural, and cognitive. In the section focusing on the analysis of the conflictual issues identified, the author adopted an eclectic stance, supporting her interpretations with selected components of the various models.

A corollary and significant element of the review of the literature concerns the "level" of sources used in the research—a subject that comes up in just about every college research methods course. In experimental and quasi-experimental studies (and other models as well), the emphasis is on primary sources. This means working from original documents or forms of sources, not secondary or tertiary levels found in the texts or articles referencing or quoting from them.

4. Operational Definitions of Key Variables

Defining a variable or concept is not to be confused with a dictionary definition—i.e., a list of synonyms. Operationalizing clarifies how the researcher is using key terminology that otherwise might have ambiguous interpretations or be unfamiliar to the reader. Within the context of a study, it explains, in concrete, descriptive terms, how a concept is to be used and how it will be measured. The definition chosen is formulated from common usage in the research literature and then adapted to meet the purposes of a particular study (Fraleigh & Hanstein, 1999; Walizer & Wiener, 1978; Simon, 1969; Kerlinger, 1973). Operationalizing exposes the researcher's intentions and establishes a common basis for understanding key concepts of the research.

As an example, in a study examining the effects of DMT with older adults who had sustained brain injuries (Berrol, Ooi, & Katz, 1997), body scheme was identified as a subset of one of four primary variables assessed. The definition included measurable items such as identification of body parts, imitation of body postures, body part awareness, and tactile awareness of body parts touched. Each of the other subsets was represented in quantifiable terms as well.

5. Issues of Validity

At the heart of all research, regardless of paradigm, is whether the research is valid. Validity refers to the inherent integrity and trustworthiness of various aspects of the research methods and results. No matter how important an idea and no matter how committed the researcher, factors violating internal validity criteria will impact the integrity of the causal relationship and as a consequence, affect the external validity of a study, meaning the ability to make inferences or to generalize the findings (Campbell & Stanley, 1966; Cook & Reichardt, 1979; Reis & Judd, 2000). As pointed out earlier, even a well designed and controlled study *does not prove* causality; replication research is necessary to augment and heighten the probability of acceptance of the research outcome.

A stunning case in point is the recent revelation of the findings of a large, well-controlled federally funded study (Women's Health Initiative) concerning the effects of Prempro™ hormone replacement therapy (HRT) in postmenopausal women. With sufficient evidence to indicate that HRT not only possessed some undetected risks, and contrary to previous research, might even increase the risk of heart attacks, the study was summarily halted. An interesting article in the *New York Times* (Kolata, 2003) questioned: "What Went Wrong?" since an earlier large, longitudinal, and well-controlled Nurses Health Study detected opposite results: that is, few risks and protection against heart attacks. So what did go wrong? Researchers concluded that there were some unanticipated factors that were not scrutinized or controlled for. Two of the issues not examined were the gender differences in etiology of heart disease and the mechanism by which estrogen is metabolized into the blood stream.

Thus, internal validity issues, which are addressed via careful design to control or rule out rival alternative hypotheses, can have a profound impact on the external validity of a study. Among the factors frequently challenging internal validity are (Kerlinger, 1973; Simon, 1969; Cook & Campbell, 1979; Campbell & Stanley, 1966; Tashakkori & Teddlie, 1998; Reis & Judd, 2000):

- Extraneous interacting events that are undetected or not accounted for;
- Changes in the sample population due to maturation as a function of time (growth, age, maturation);
- Small sample size;
- An unrepresentative sample of the population under study;
- Lack of a control group for comparison of any changes that might be revealed;
- Any number of unaccounted-for extraneous factors such as competing activities or new medications;
- The control group receives only the posttest, meaning that there is no way to insure that the groups were initially comparable—equivalent to comparing apples and oranges;
- Uncontrolled differences (variables) between or among sample groups;
- Sample attrition leading to an incomplete data set that might skew comparability of groups;
- Questionable validity of the test measures employed;
- Questionable choice of statistical procedures (i.e., tests to determine statistical significance);
- Subjectivity of testers or raters regarding test administration (i.e., one rater might be an easy scorer, another a tough scorer, or the tester might harbor biases toward the subject that could result in a higher or lower grade (i.e., halo effect);
- Significant changes may be influenced by the effect of a particular therapist on a group and/or the act of being a participant in a study (i.e., Hawthorne effect).

Kerlinger (1973) maintains that the degree to which researchers can have confidence in the outcome of a study is consonant with the degree to which they are able to control internal validity issues.

6. Methods and Procedures

Here begins the true heart of the research inquiry: sample selection and research design; choice of measurement tools and statistical analysis; and intervention procedures (Fraleigh & Harnstein, 1999). Aspects of the research process are amplified as follows.

6.1. Sample Selection. Prior to sample selection, there is a critical preliminary step to be carried out: obtaining informed consent. Each institution that oversees research has in place an Institutional Review Board (IRB) that approves any research involving human subjects. The IRB oversees ethical concerns, primarily the protection of individuals from undue risk or harm and the assurance of anonymity. Before beginning the investigation, the researcher must apply to the IRB for their required protocols. The materials submitted for review commonly include details about the research design and the procedures (intervention) relative to the human subjects. IRB approval is necessary before the project can be undertaken. Once approval is obtained, the next step may begin.

Sample selection is contingent upon receiving informed consent from each potential participant. Sample refers to the group of individuals who participate in a research study. Since it's impossible to carry out a study with all members of a particular population, the sample represents a subset of that universe. It could be children with autism, teenage girls with identified eating disorders, young adults who are drug abusers, or older adults with Alzheimer's disease—in other words, any group that the researcher wishes to investigate. The nature of the study will help determine how and from where the sample will be culled.

In the study cited earlier (examining the effect of DMT with older adults with brain injury), two of the primary criteria for participation were age and type of disability. Individuals had to be at least 60 years old, and to have sustained some type of nonprogressive neurotrauma such as stroke, traumatic brain injury, or cerebral aneurysm. Likewise, individuals had to be able to function in a group situation regardless of cognitive or communicative deficits resulting from the neurotrauma. Excluded from this study were persons diagnosed with progressive dementias such as Alzheimer's disease, or "who are otherwise unable to participate in a group" (Berrol, Ooi, & Katz, 1997, p. 138). Note that criteria for both inclusion and exclusion were delineated.

6.2. Research Methods. Various research designs are employed in experimental investigations. One of the most common is the comparison of two or more groups before and after some experimental condition is implemented. Under ideal conditions individuals are randomly assigned to the sample groups. Participants of the experimental group are exposed to the special condition while controls do not receive any special treatment or may receive an alternative intervention. Groups are tested before and after the intervention to discern whether the special condition had an impact on the experimental subjects (Walizer & Wienir, 1978).

Random group assignment connotes a method in which each subject has an equal chance of being placed in either the experimental or control group(s). Large samples help factor out demographic issues that could potentially skew the outcome of the research, variables such as gender, age, socio-economic level, intelligence, ethnicity, and education. If differences between groups are discerned during pretests on baseline measures, special techniques, such as matching groups or statistically neutralizing the differences, are used to compensate for this problem (Walizer & Wienir, 1978). In the study referenced above (Berrol, Ooi, & Katz, 1997), random assignment of subjects to groups was not possible because of patient scheduling problems within some of the rehabilitation facilities involved in the project. Therefore the statistical procedure of analysis of covariance was employed to adjust for demographic differences.

Kerlinger (1973) contends that a good research design follows what he terms the "Maxmincon Principle" (p. 306). This refers to three basic premises that can be summarized as follows:

1. First, if a study compares two groups exposed to two different experimental conditions (e.g., an independent variable with two levels such as dance/movement therapy and dance classes), it is important to *maximize* the differences between the two to allow for the predicted effect (on the dependent variable) to emerge. If the two conditions are not sufficiently different, the effect may be obscured.

2. Second, it's necessary to *minimize* or control "error variance," depicted as "random, fluctuations or extraneous factors" which are not the focus of the study but which may mask its outcome. Error variance may be likened to a child with an attention deficit disorder who is hypersensitive to sound and can't filter out extraneous auditory background to attend what is being said. Kerlinger informs that the larger the sample group, the smaller the random error variance. Measurement error is another common source of error variance (see Cruz & Koch in this text).

3. The final premise deals with *control* of extraneous variables, that is, eliminating or neutralizing unwanted interference that may skew the experimental effect—a serious internal validity issue. Differences in age, gender, and socioeconomic level are but a few of the potentially problematic factors common in many studies. In the study cited earlier regarding the impact of DMT on older individuals (Berrol, Ooi, & Katz, 1997), one potential source of an unwanted variance was "time," that is, whether the duration of time between the occurrence of the neurotrauma (shorter versus longer) and the start of the intervention had a biasing impact on the effect of the treatment. The statistical analytic procedure conducted to discern a possible interaction revealed no significant effect based on the "time" variable.

Kerlinger views the Maxmincon Principle as essential to creating a design that helps the researcher rule out alternative causal explanations or predictors.

6.3. Measurement Instrument. Typically in experimental designs, pre- and posttests measuring selected dependent variables are administered to the sample groups to discern whether meaningful differences between or among them can be attributed to an intervention (independent variable). Thus the integrity of instruments chosen to measure dependent variables is a vital component of the validity of a study. Cruz and Koch (see Chapter 4 in this text on validity and reliability) clearly explain the issues involved in test validity and their critical role in research.

One of the first considerations of choosing measures is the appropriateness and sensitivity of the instrument relative to the premises of the research variables. The researcher justifies the use of measurements chosen by a careful review of reported validity and reliability data. Well designed, standardized test instruments chronicle, in detail, information regarding the various stages of a test's development, including validity and reliability data.

In a research project examining the effects of DMT on first-grade children with learning and perceptual motor problems (Berrol, 1984), one of the dependent variables was hyperactivity. The Children's Checking, the instrument administered to measure this variable, was deemed an appropriate measure because it was purported to be a research tool specifically "developed to assess hyperactive children whose problems are associated with learning disorders" (Margolis, 1972, p. 64). Likewise, Berrol supported this selection with credible validity and reliability data reported by the test developer.

On the other hand, in the study reporting the effects of DMT with older individuals who had sustained brain injuries (Berrol, Ooi, & Katz, 1997), the instrument used to measure depression was found to be inappropriate for the sample group. When posttest findings failed to detect significant differences between the experimental and control groups on this variable, the researchers carefully reviewed the test manual regarding the purported intention of the scale as well as its design. They noted that it was developed as a basic screening tool to identify patients who were depressed. The researchers concluded that although the depression scale may have been a useful screening tool, it was not sufficiently discriminating for the purposes of the study.

6.4. Data Collection and Analysis. In quantitative research, both descriptive data—information regarding the demographics[2] of the samples—and data

---

[2] Demographic data provide information about the characteristics of a group that may have an effect on the variables under review such as age, level of education, gender, ethnicity, and socio-economic group. For example, age and gender might affect the level of physical fitness of a group so it would be important to assess the relationship between the two before treatment begins to adjust for these factors. Demographics also play an important part in survey research.

[3] It is beyond the scope of this paper to discuss the various statistical procedures employed in quantitative designs. Highly sophisticated statistical computer programs can be run to calculate and analyze the different data sets.

related to the independent and dependent variables are gathered and collated. Appropriate statistical procedures[3] are selected and conducted to analyze both types of data. The data are statistically analyzed in different ways appropriate to the design of the research. Often, designs that compare two or more groups allow researchers to examine mean score changes between or among the groups.

6.5. Intervention. A detailed description of the intervention—design, process, and theoretical underpinnings—is an important feature of a research proposal and postresearch review. Earlier, in this chapter, theoretical constructs and operational definitions were identified as two key substrates of research inquiry. In effect, the procedures for the experimental condition are driven by these phenomena or may be conceived as extensions of them. Dance/movement therapists have only to review the application of the American Dance Therapy Association (ADTA) for ADTR registry to find that applicants are asked to identify and discuss the theoretical bases of their clinical practices as well as to provide examples of how these theories are incorporated into their clinical practices.

To demonstrate how a theoretically driven intervention might be constructed, the research exploring the effects of DMT with first-grade children displaying learning and perceptual motor problems will be used again (Berrol, 1984). The DMT intervention was guided by two developmental models: ontogenesis—the "wired-in" process of growth and maturation in human development (the theories of A. Jean Ayres, Newell Kephart, and Marian Frostig); and child development (the theories of Jean Piaget and Eric Erikson). These sources helped articulate developmental constructs used to shape the goals of the DMT intervention—i.e., the areas of emphasis in the DMT sessions—and guide the selection of measurement instruments. The primary targets of therapy were identified as balance and posture, body image, visual perception, visual-motor integration, hyperactivity, sensory-motor discrimination, and cognition. These variables were operationally defined. The intervention was structured within the framework of age appropriate developmental expectations. Fundamental patterns of locomotor and nonlocomotor movement were explored in concert with the elements of time, space, weight, and flow. The DMT sessions incorporated props, story telling, mirroring, musical instruments, et cetera. The specific details of the intervention in relation to the underlying theoretical models and stated goals were described.

Another important component of treatment is the "dose" needed to get an effect, that is, the total time span of the treatment and the number of sessions and/or hours per week (see also Chapter 10 in this volume). The study referred to above spanned thirteen weeks and each of the two groups receiving treatment interventions (Experimental group—DMT, described above, and Comparison group—sensory integration) participated in three thirty-minute sessions a week (i.e., thirty-nine sessions).

7. Results

The research design just presented is an example of a study in which both the treatment and the comparison control group were tested on the dependent variables before the intervention began and then after completion of the treatment. The next step in this type of research is the analysis of differences between pre- and posttest scores to discern whether statistically significant differences are registered that can be attributed to the experimental condition. Results are based on empirical (observable) and quantifiable data that are statistically analyzed. Ultimately it is the statistical magnitude of differences between scores on variables that will determine the outcome of the predictions.

Depending on the statistical design, different combinations of factors may be isolated, paired, or grouped for comparative analysis. The findings of the different statistical analyses are reported and discussed. Whether a directional or nondirectional research hypothesis was formulated, the researcher will discuss results within that framework, stating whether or not the null hypothesis can be rejected.

8. Interpreting Results and Making Inferences

When research is in the form of a thesis, dissertation, or publication, results and their implications are presented in a discussion format. Creative and thought provoking, this narrative provides the researcher with the opportunity to synthesize the disparate elements of the research into a comprehensible whole, one of the most stimulating aspects of the process. It involves making sense of the outcomes, interpreting what they mean, and using "informed intuiting," or reasoning why they might have occurred. Importantly, the discussion is keyed to the theoretical constructs on which the research is predicated. In addition, the researcher shares insights gleaned or inferences drawn that might augment and enhance the theoretical concepts. Coming full circle, the researcher crystallizes and intertwines the premises and goals of the study with its outcome, clearly explicating the relationships between and/or among them.

Another aspect of the discussion is the identification of the study's weakness and limitations, i.e., elements that impact on the validity and outcome. Predictability and generalizability (external validity) will be circumscribed by the integrity of the research with respect to the robustness of its internal validity.

9. Conclusion

The final leg of the research journey is simply a brief overview of the project. Aspects of the research literature may be incorporated, that is, the referencing of similar studies, comparing and contrasting them to the inquiry under review. In addition, the closing section generally includes suggestions for future research and some reflections on how the investigation amplifies or deepens the existing body of knowledge.

ALTERNATIVES TO EXPERIMENTAL DESIGNS IN SCIENTIFIC RESEARCH

The remainder of the chapter will briefly review some alternative options to the experimental and quasi-experimental methods already discussed. Although they broaden the parameters of inquiry with respect to purpose and design, these alternatives remain in the domain of quantitative or scientific research. Nevertheless, it's important to understand that most research inquiry may be constructed as either qualitative or quantitative studies or as a combination of the two (see Chapter 12 in this text, "How to Mix Quantitative and Qualitative Methods in a Dance/Movement Therapy Research Project").

Descriptive Research: Observation and Survey Methods

Defined as studies that identify and describe specific characteristics of various types of phenomena, descriptive research can generally be dichotomized into observation and survey methods. Descriptive studies do not involve hypothesis testing of cause-effect relationships, evaluating the effectiveness of treatment interventions, or measurement instruments (Borg, Gall, & Gall, 1993; Simon, 1969). Rather, descriptive studies are primarily concerned with finding out "what is." Correlational studies are a variant of descriptive research in which the focus is on discovering and clarifying the relationships and the magnitude of relationships between or among variables (Borg & Gall, 1979).

Observation Research

As the name implies, this mode of research is the direct observational study of individuals or groups under varying conditions, depending on the purpose of the research. Anthropologic research and case study research are typically classified as descriptive forms, but observational studies are not limited to these methods. Observational studies are defined by the collection of data on some existing persons or group of individuals who are of interest to the researcher. Jean Piaget is a prime example of a researcher who based his theories of cognitive development on meticulous and well documented longitudinal observations of his daughters Jacqueline and Lucienne, and son Laurent. Many well established theoretical constructs are based on observational research, such as those of Sigmund Freud (psychological development), Erik Erikson (psychosocial development), and Lawrence Kohlberg (moral development).

Sometimes, descriptive research using narrative data designed to identify, describe, and interpret the behavioral characteristics of particular individuals, groups, or cultures, is analyzed via the method known as content or interpretive analysis. However, there are instances in which an observation is configured for quantitative measurement. Lausberg (1998), for example, conducted a study to examine whether the motility patterns of two groups with different forms of eating disorders, anorexia nervosa and bulimia nervosa, would be diagnostically discernable. Selected parameters of Laban Movement Analysis (LMA), a system of movement observation familiar to most dance/movement therapists, were employed to establish the movement variables to be scrutinized, quantified, and statistically analyzed for measurement purposes. The chapters in this text focusing on case study research (Chaiklin & Chaiklin) and qualitative methods (Forinash) address various procedures for conducting descriptive research and analyzing narrative data.

Survey Research

Alternatively referred to as questionnaires, surveys are created to examine various sample groups on a spectrum of issues and topics, be they personal behaviors, habits, opinions, feelings, attitudes—just about anything (Borg & Gall, 1979; Walizer & Wienir, 1978). Most people have had experiences with surveys, whether public opinion polls on political issues, commercial products, or health issues; the list is endless. It is likely that most dance therapists are familiar with some sort of discipline-related survey whether as graduate students or clinicians gathering data for a project, or the alternative, providing data for someone else's questionnaire. Although survey inquiries can vary in methodological design, in this chapter this approach is examined within the context of descriptive research.

A preponderance of surveys are created to obtain quantifiable data; nevertheless, some are devised for narrative responses or include narrative components that can be content analyzed to extrapolate common trends or patterns. On the other hand, the narrative responses may be coded to enable quantitative examination. Surveys constructed for a sample geared to a particular population may be conducted via telephone or personal interview, postal or electronic mail.

When quantified, questions are grouped categorically to facilitate conversion to numerical values. The data are computed as frequencies to establish how the responses to the various questions are distributed among the sample group. Census taking is an ubiquitous example of a descriptive survey (Isaac & Michael, 1981; Borg & Gall, 1979).

Formatting the Questions. In addition to different types of surveys, there are different options for formatting questions. Some are posited as discrete "Yes" or "No" queries: "Do you smoke?" "Have you ever been hospitalized?"

Many descriptive surveys incorporate multiple choice items. When collecting demographic data, some questions—for example, age, gender, type of employment, and level of education—can be answered by marking the given choice that best applies. Obviously, the number of options depends on the specific question. For instance, a question such as "What is your marital status?" might offer the following four options: "single, married, divorced, widowed." A question about an individual's age might be grouped into age ranges: □ 20–29; □ 30–39; □ 40–49.

A common format devised for attitude surveys is the Likert-type scale, offering a selection of options to allow for serial rankings. Responses are numerically ranked from high to low (or vice versa) and easily tabulated. A sample of this type of format is displayed in Figure 3-1.

Figure 3-1   Example of Likert-type Survey Item

Statement:

DMT should be included in special education legislation as a supplemental service

Answers might be worded and scored as follows:

4	3	2	1	0
□ *Strongly agree*	□ *Somewhat agree*	□ *Somewhat disagree*	□ *Strongly disagree*	□ *No opinion*

Recently, a survey developed by the ADTA Research Committee was conducted to determine the attitudes and interests of ADTA members concerning research. It was sent via mail to all members of the ADTA. Results reported in the *American Journal of Dance Therapy* (Cruz & Hervey, 2001) included demographic information in addition to research background and experience. The data were primarily reported as percentages. For instance, one of the findings regarding age distributions revealed that 42 percent of the respondents were between ages forty and forty-nine years; another of the findings indicated that 60 percent of the respondents' clinical work included psychiatric cases.

Questions configured to be answered as *Yes* or *No* were, similarly, converted to percentages. One of the questions inquired whether the therapist had ever "sent a research article to the journal?" The authors reported that 22 percent of the respondents had and 78 percent had not. Part 2 of the questionnaire shifted to a narrative-style inquiry, probing feelings about doing research, and attitudes about the value of research. The authors provided a narrative summary of and commentary on these findings.

Validity Issues in Survey Research. According to various authors, good surveys are very difficult to design and quite vulnerable to all sorts of difficulties (Borg, Gall, & Gall, 1993; Walizer & Wienir, 1978; Simon, 1969;
Kerlinger, 1973). While there is common acknowledgment of the value of
this type of inquiry, there is also recognition of the potential for investigator bias. Simply the way a question is posed can tweak the response.
Consider public opinion polls commonly generated in the political arena
where the type of questions asked and the phrasing used may be skewed to
lead to a particular type of response. Authors commenting on this problem
conclude that it is the responsibility of researchers formulating surveys to
strive to create neutral, bias free instruments.

On the other hand, there is no foolproof mechanism to either insure or
determine the veracity of an individual's answer. Highly subjective in nature,
respondents may be reluctant to reveal their true opinions, thoughts, feelings, or beliefs, regardless of the reason (Borg & Gall, 1979). Any self-
reporting procedure has the potential for a large margin of error. Even
when a researcher employs or modifies existing surveys, validity issues must
be given careful consideration. Whether developed by the researcher or
using an extant instrument, validity warrants mindful scrutiny. Various
aspects of validity were touched upon earlier in this chapter.

Some additional concerns related to survey research are nonresponse
bias, and errors in defining and sampling the population (Smith & Glass,
1987). Pointing out this type of problem, Cruz and Hervey (2001) stated,
"Research evidence suggests that responders may be different from nonre-
spondents on characteristics as varied as level of education and interest in
the topic (Rosenthal & Rosnow, 1975). In addition, response rates lower
than 20 percent can decrease the precision of sample estimates calculated
from the data (Cochran, 1977)" (p. 108). While there are techniques to
address nonresponse bias such as in-person interviews or direct phone
administration, surveys may likewise be associated with other problems such
as social desirability concerns that color the responses to questions.
Reasonable care should be taken when planning and interpreting survey
research to address these inherent problems.

Historical Inquiry

Learning about and gaining insights into the past provides a context for
and gateway into the present. Historical inquiry is a significant key to understanding our world and to creating our personal worldview. Historical
research is undertaken to objectively and accurately trace and reconstruct
events, developments, or experiences of past periods. Findings are interpreted on the basis of documented evidence (Borg, Gall, & Gall, 1993;
Kerlinger, 1973). The researcher conducts a systematic examination of
sources, including literature, archival material, and artifacts, plus other rel-

evant documentation concerning specific questions or hypotheses (Isaac & Michael, 1981; Kerlinger, 1973; Borg & Gall, 1993).

A rule of thumb for historical investigation is the use of primary sources (Borg, Gall, & Gall, 1993; Kerlinger, 1973; Hanstein, 1999a). This means gathering authentic data, specifically from those who created them or witnesses who observed, participated in, and/or documented them in some form. A case in point might be someone researching the formative years of modern dance. One viable source might be newspapers of that era containing accounts of and reviews written about (or by) the choreographers and their works. *Dance Observer*, a newsletter published during that period, specialized in reviews, commentary, and information about the world of modern dance. Archived in various university and performing arts libraries, this chronicle would be a valid primary source.

Secondary sources, based on information derived from the original, are acceptable when original documents are no longer available. Tertiary sources refer to information cited from secondary levels—i.e., two steps beyond the original (Hanstein, 1999b). Problems with secondary and tertiary sources include possible distortions or misinterpretations, the particular spin the respective researcher might incorporate into his/her writing, or the extrapolation of a segment taken out of context and viewed with a different lens. The main issue with secondary or tertiary sources is the accuracy of the content (Borg & Gall, 1979; Kerlinger, 1973). Like the game of telephone, the further removed from the source, the greater the degree of transmutation or misrepresentation.

Researching first-level sources is possible when documents are available and accessible. A feasible topic might include the development of DMT in the United States, or the pioneers of DMT and their specific contributions. *The Life and Work of Marian Chace* (Sandel, Chaiklin, & Lohn, 1993) contains a number of chapters authored by individuals who trained and/or worked with Marian Chace. These individuals would be considered authentic sources.

On the other hand, for many dance/movement therapists and graduate students, the requisite of using primary sources may be beyond the realm of possibility, especially when a project incorporates anthropological data. Some years ago, a DMT graduate student working on her thesis investigated the use of the circle in group therapy. A survey of dance/movement therapists to ascertain how/when/why they utilized the circle in sessions propelled the student into an in-depth examination of the universal symbolism of the circle. In addition, the student researched the use and significance of the circle in various early cultures—a dip into the anthropologic realm. In this case, delving into the archetypal meanings and implications of the circle necessitated the use of secondary and tertiary sources.

CONCLUSION

This chapter concentrated on the conceptual framework and methods of experimental research, a form grounded in deductive reasoning and most closely associated with quantitative methods. Experimental and quasi-experimental designs were represented and explained, including related issues of validity and reliability. Definitions of essential research factors were provided throughout. The basic components and process of designing quantitative research were explained and in many instances supplemented by relevant examples to assist the reader in concretizing the information. Alternative options within the scientific mode of inquiry, survey and historical research, were reviewed to offer a more comprehensive view of the spectrum of experimental research approaches than might otherwise be considered.

Even within the scientific realm, often perceived by dance/movement therapists as unapproachable, uninviting, and/or inappropriate for the creative arts, there is really no glass ceiling regarding the potential for exploration, discovery, and interpretation. An individual's imagination or resourcefulness need not be circumscribed by the form of the inquiry. Ultimately, the mode undertaken should be contingent upon the paradigm or paradigms (i.e., mixed methods) best suited to answer the research questions posed and to meet the overarching goals of the research. The goodness of fit is the primary consideration.

REFERENCES

Aldridge, D., & Aldridge, G. (1996). A personal construct methodology for validating subjectivity in qualitative research. *The Arts in Psychotherapy, 23*(3), 225–236.

Berrol, C. F. (1984). The effects of two movement therapy approaches on selected academic, physical and socio-behavioral measures of first grade children with learning and perceptual-motor problems. *American Journal of Dance Therapy, 7*, 32–48.

Berrol, C. F., Ooi, W. L., & Katz, S. S. (1997). Dance/movement therapy with older adults who have sustained neurological insult: A demonstration project. *American Journal of Dance Therapy, 19*(2), 135–160.

Borg, W. R., & Gall, M. D. (1979). *Educational research: An introduction* (3rd ed.). New York: Longman.

Borg, W. R., Gall, J. P., & Gall, M. D. (1993). *Applying educational research: A practical guide* (3rd ed.). New York: Longman.

Campbell, D. T., & Stanley, J. C. (1966). *Experimental and quasi-experimental designs for research.* Chicago, IL: Rand McNally.

Chatfield, S. J. (1999). Scientific exploration in dance. In S. Horton Fraleigh & P. Hanstein (Eds.), *Researching dance: Evolving modes of inquiry* (pp. 124–162). Pittsburgh, PA: University of Pittsburgh Press.

Cook, T. D., & Campbell, D. T. (1979). *Quasi-experimentation: Design & analysis issues for field settings.* Chicago, IL: Rand McNally College Publishing Co.

Cook, T. D., & Reichardt, C. S. (Eds.). (1979). *Qualitative and quantitative methods in evaluation research.* Beverly Hills, CA: Sage.

Cresswell, J. W. (1994). *Research design: Qualitative and quantitative approaches.* Thousand Oaks, CA: Sage.

Cruz, R., & Hervey, L. (2001). The American Dance Therapy Association research survey. *American Journal of Dance Therapy, 23*(2), 89–118.

Erikson, E. (1963). Childhood and society. New York: W.W. Norton.

Feder, B., & Feder, E. (1998). *The art and science of evaluation in the arts therapies.* Springfield, IL: Charles C Thomas.

Forinash, M. (1995). Phenomenological research. In B. L.Wheeler (Ed.), *Music therapy research: quantitative and qualitative perspectives* (pp. 368–387). Phoenixville, PA: Barcelona Publishers.

Fraleigh, S. H., & Hanstein, P. (Eds.). (1999). *Researching dance: Evolving modes of inquiry.* Pittsburgh, PA: University of Pittsburgh Press.

Gantt, L. M. (1998). A discussion of art therapy as a science. *Art Therapy, 15*(1), 3–12.

Green, J., & Horton, S. W. (1999). Postpositivist research in dance. In S. H. Fraleigh & P. Hanstein (Eds.), *Researching dance: Evolving modes of inquiry* (pp. 91–123). Pittsburgh, PA: University of Pittsburgh Press.

Guralnik, D. B. (Ed.). (1992). *Webster's new world dictionary of the American language.* New York: Warner Brooks.

Hanstein, P. (1999a). From idea to research proposal: Balancing the systematic and serendipitous. In S. H. Fraleigh & P. Hanstein (Eds.), *Researching dance: Evolving modes of inquiry* (pp. 22–61). Pittsburgh, PA: University of Pittsburgh Press.

Hanstein, P. (1999b). Models and metaphors: Theory making and the creation of new knowledge. In S. H. Fraleigh & P. Hanstein (Eds.), *Researching dance: Evolving modes of inquiry* (pp. 62–90). Pittsburgh, PA: University of Pittsburgh Press.

Isaac, S., & Michael, W. B. (1981). *Handbook in research and evaluation* (2nd ed.). San Diego, CA: Robert R. Knapp.

Kerlinger, F. (1973). *Foundations of behavioral research* (2nd ed.). New York: Holt, Rinehart and Winston.

Kolata, G. (April 22, 2003). Hormone studies: What went wrong? *The New York Times,* pp. D1, D6.

Lausberg, H. (1998). Does movement behavior have differential diagnostic potential? Discussion of a controlled study on patients with anorexia nervosa and bulimia. *American Journal of Dance Therapy, 20*(2), 85–99.

Margolis, J. S. (1972). *Academic correlates of sustained attention.* Unpublished Doctoral Dissertation, University of California, Los Angeles.

McNiff, S. A. (1987). Research and scholarship in the creative arts therapies. *The Arts in Psychotherapy, 14*(4), 285–292.

Neuman, I., & Benz, C. R. (1998). *Qualitative-quantitative research methodology: Exploring the interactive continuum.* Carbondale, IL: Southern Illinois University Press.

Politsky, R. H. (1995). Toward a typology of research in the creative arts therapies. *The Arts in Psychotherapy, 22*(4), 307–314.

Rehavia-Hanauer, D. (2003). Identifying conflicts of anorexia nervosa as manifested in the art therapy process. *The Arts in Psychotherapy, 30*(3), 137–149.

Reis, H. T., & Judd, C. M. (2000). *Handbook of research methods in social and personality psychology.* New York: Cambridge University Press.

Sandel, S. L., Chaiklin, S., & Lohn, A. (Eds.). (1993). *Foundations of dance movement therapy: The life and work of Marian Chace.* Columbia, MD: The Marian Chace Memorial Fund.

Simon, J. L. (1969). *Basic research in social science: The art of empirical research.* New York: Random House.

Smith, M. L., & Glass, G. V. (1987). *Research and evaluation in education and the social sciences.* Boston: Allyn and Bacon.

Stewart, C. *The symbolic impetus: How creative fantasy motivates development.* New York: Free Association Books.

Tashakkori, A., & Teddlie, C. (1998). *Mixed methodology: Combining qualitative and quantitative approaches* (Vol. 46). Thousand Oaks, CA: Sage.

Walizer, M. H., & Wienir, P. L. (1978). *Research methods and analysis: Searching for relationships.* New York: Harper & Row.

Chapter 4

ISSUES OF VALIDITY AND RELIABILITY IN THE USE OF MOVEMENT OBSERVATIONS AND SCALES

ROBYN FLAUM CRUZ AND SABINE C. KOCH

Whether for diagnostic purposes or intervention, dance/movement therapists use movement observations to provide important data for the practice of dance/movement therapy (DMT). Regardless of the particular approach within DMT, observing clients' movements and changes in movement create the element that makes DMT unique among the psychotherapies. This chapter gives guidelines to using observational data in research studies of dance/movement therapy that can also be applied to movement observation used in clinical practice. Because of the importance of movement observations to DMT work, and the availability of many superior treatments of reliability and validity with respect to paper and pencil tests or other types of scales used in research (see for example, Feder & Feder, 1998; Anastasi, 1988), our discussion will focus specifically on validity and reliability for observational data. We give particular attention to the different types of observational data, flaws and advantages related to using movement observations, and the criteria that need to be established for scientific credibility of observations—validity and reliability. Examples based on Laban Movement Analysis (1947, 1974, 1980), the Kestenberg Movement Profile (KMP; Kestenberg, 1975), and the Movement Psychodiagnostic Inventory (MPI; Davis, 1991) will be introduced as we explore the issues of validity and reliability of movement observations and scales, and we include a simple "how-to" example for calculating an index of rater agreement that we hope will be helpful to clinicians and researchers.

What does it really mean to speak of the validity and reliability of movement observations and scales? In simple terms, *validity* is the degree to which an observation scale measures what it is supposed to measure (precision), while *reliability* is defined as the consistency or accuracy of the scores that result from the observation measurement process. These terms relate to important arguments that DMT researchers and clinicians want to make about the truthfulness of their observations. For example, based on clinical observation, a dance/movement therapist might wish to examine if people with anxiety disorders display a unique set of movement characteristics. To address validity, one would need to specify what these movement characteristics are, and find a movement observation scale that allows these exact movement features to be measured. To address reliability, one would need to demonstrate that independent observers can rate these features with similar accuracy. Yet, once the process of establishing arguments for the validity and reliability of observations is begun, it is also possible to begin to examine interesting relationships between observations and other phenomena which can be communicated to colleagues in DMT and other professions. Eventually, this information can be used to improve the quality of the treatment that dance/movement therapists offer. We start our in-depth look at validity and reliability by first considering the nature of movement observation.

MOVEMENT OBSERVATION

Movement observation, like any type of observation, has a subjective component. Perception can be compromised by selectivity, prior knowledge, interpretation, and other factors. Constructionist views assume that there is no objective reality; that what is seen, perceived, and described is always dependent on the observer (see for example, Gergen, 1985). This constructive nature of observations was described by Gestalt psychologists at the beginning of the twentieth century. They contended that humans tend to complement perceptual patterns following certain rules, such as the "good Gestalt" (Koffka, 1935; Köhler, 1924/33). This means that humans are inclined to change patterns to fit what they are used to seeing or what they expect to see. So how can criteria for scientific observation be established?

First, there is a need to distinguish perception and description. The gap between what humans perceive and what they can describe is especially large in movement observation. Everyday language provides only a limited vocabulary for movement description, and using this limited means can compromise the communication of the movement phenomena perceived. The fleeting nature of motion and the limited capacities of the perceptual system are additional obstacles to reliable observation and description. Laban (1947/1974, 1980) created a specialized language to describe the visible dynamics of movement that enables those who use it to more quickly grasp what is seen in motion and communicate it to others more effectively, thus laying the groundwork for a scientific means of using movement observations in research. His system merely sets the stage—there still must be attempts to control individual tendencies toward selectivity in observing, or the subjectivity of perception. It is attempts to use systems such as Laban's to decode movement in controlled ways that allow movement observations to be more scientific.

By scientific, we mean that observations differ from everyday observations in specific ways. Scientific observation is an intentional, attention-selective way of perceiving (Graumann, 1966). Certain specific aspects are focused on at the cost of other aspects, and efforts are made to address objectivity by using constructs and definitions to define the focus of the observation. Scientific, as opposed to everyday, observation is approached in a planful and selective way, determined by a searching attitude, and directed towards analysis and assessment of well defined constructs. In addition, scientific observations are assessed in terms of the extent to which they satisfy criteria such as reliability and validity. In the following sections, we discuss these concepts about how observations, such as the clinical observations made in DMT work, can be transformed into scientific observations.

Types of Observations

The key to defining what constitutes scientific observations is that they must be systematic. Making observations of the same client at the same set time points during treatment is a form of being systematic. Making observations of the same client only on days when the therapist thinks they might see a change is not being systematic. Taking the time to systematically note and document what is seen in movement allows clinicians to collect valuable data for treatment intervention. Systematic observation can be structured, meaning that observation is done with explicit predefined categories, or unstructured, meaning that observation is done without explicit predefined categories. Structured and unstructured observation can also be either participatory, passive participatory, or nonparticipatory, indicating the degree of psychological distance to the object under investigation. In DMT groups an observer can be an active participant (such as the therapist), a passive participant sitting in one corner of the room making notes, or he or she can be nonparticipatory by just observing a videotape of a DMT session. Structured and unstructured observations can be further classified as: (a) overt or covert, indicating whether the observed persons know that they are observed; (b) mediated by technical means such as videotape or nonmediated; or (c) performed in the laboratory or the field, indicating whether the setting is natural or artificial. Many movement observation scales are designed for a particular type of observation context. For example, the Movement Psychodiagnostic Inventory (MPI; Davis, 1991) is designed for continuous observing and recording of a videotaped, one-on-one clinical interview situation where the clinician is not the researcher, so it can be defined as structured, nonparticipatory, overt, mediated, and field study. Similarly, the Kestenberg Movement Profile (KMP; Kestenberg, 1975) is most commonly used with videos of patients, and thus is structured, nonparticipatory, overt, mediated, and laboratory or field study depending on the setting. As with other types of movement observation scales, both of these systems can also be used less formally in clinical practice.

Movement Observation Coding Systems

In clinical practice and research dance/movement therapists sometimes work with established coding systems like the KMP and MPI, but what if one were to build a coding system of his or her own? There would be many decisions to be made, such as deciding on the context for observation, the observational units of time, and what types of and how many categories of movement behavior one expects to be able to note. This last element may be more important than it seems at first glance. Psychologists have found that because of humans' limited cognitive capacity, most people cannot observe more than five categories with two subcategories at a time (Amelang & Zielinski, 1997). If an individual is creating his or her own system, this rule of thumb should probably be considered. Part of the complexity of using the KMP and the MPI is that the task demand placed on the rater is intensive, even after the long and rigorous process of rater training is completed. While an existing coding system might fit one's needs, sometimes the DMT researcher or clinician has a specific need that requires constructing a system. This was the situation when Berrol and Katz developed the Functional Assessment of Movement and Perception and used it in their study of DMT for older adults with neurological impairments (Berrol & Katz, 1990, 1993; Berrol, Ooi, & Katz, 1997). They created and refined a tool for their specific purpose and needs.

Another example is the work of Goodman (1991), who was interested in the stylistic differences in movement patterns for boys with and without hyperactivity. The coding system she devised was elegant and efficient; boys in the study were observed for four movement features: quickness, strength, intensity, and unexpected transition. Rater training used three standard but good methods: a descriptive manual, guided observations, and actual rating practice. The extent to which the raters agreed in their ratings of the boys using the coding system was .70 or better, and the raters were college students without previous movement observation experience. While there might have been additional movement features that could have been included, paring the coding system down to four well-defined features was efficient and effective; unskilled raters were used and results of the study were informative. Careful, focused planning is probably the most important aspect of developing a coding scheme. For a good description of the process and intricacies of defining a coding system, we suggest Davis (1987). Sometimes, it may seem easier to put fragments of others' coding schemes together—a few items from this one and a few from that one. We advise against this "soup pot" method because it can prevent the dance/movement therapist from thoroughly thinking through the movement features that are most important to his or her purpose. While it's more time consuming to construct one's own, the scheme produced through thoughtful consideration is likely to be better and have better validity than one cobbled together quickly.

Participant Effects and Context Considerations

There are important considerations whenever movement observation will be used concerning who is observed and the circumstances of the observation context. It is important to consider the conditions for the observation because the conditions need to be the same for every participant. Not surprisingly, most people want to be "at their best" when someone is watching them, whether the observer is in the room or will watch on videotape at a later time. *Social desirability* is the term used to describe this human phenomenon. If observations are videotaped, attention to the length of the observation period can assist the researcher in obtaining footage in which participants have relaxed, adjusted to the presence of the camera, or even forgotten about the camera. If the length of the original observation is a standard amount of time, one can choose to take a middle or later portion of the observation time to control for the nervousness or social desirability factor of participants. It is also possible to have participants engaged in conversation or another type of activity to increase their naturalness. This type of attention to the context of the observation is relevant to getting a good sample of the desired movement behavior. While the naturalness of the participants is important in sampling movement features, it is also important to make sure that raters have unobstructed views of the person they are rating. When videotaping, artifacts can be introduced by the camera angle; a feature may not be rated if raters cannot see the body parts where it is taking place. Similarly, a two-dimensional picture from videotape can sometimes lead to difficulties in identifying movement in one of the three planes (see Wallbott, 1982). The appropriate time frame and time units for reliable observation also have to be planned. Some movement features may have different baseline frequencies that are affected by the time frame of the observation. A feature may not be observed because there was not enough time for it to appear. This is unfortunately an issue that has not often been addressed with respect to movement observation systems. Establishment of an observation time frame and frequency norms for scales like the KMP are needed. While a minimal time frame of ten minutes per observation is recommended for the KMP, there is no empirical documentation of this time frame, rather it is simply assumed that there will be enough repetition to identify behavioral patterns and frequencies. For some types of movement observation, one may be interested in sequential aspects or contingencies in movement rather than frequencies. In this case, time can be considered, for example, by using pattern analysis software (e.g., THEME, Magnusson, 2000).

Observer Effects and Bias

There are several types of faulty observer or rater response tendencies that cause observations to be biased, meaning consistently or systematically in error. *Halo effects* describe a rater's tendency to base ratings on a general overall impression rather than occurrence of the actual characteristics that are supposed to be rated (Saal, Downey, & Lahey, 1980). For example, imagine if one of Goodman's (1991) raters awarded fewer ratings of quickness, strength, intensity, and unexpected transition to the boys who had blue eyes than those with other eye colors. This rater would be basing ratings on eye color rather than the movement characteristics as defined in the coding system. While this rater might not have substantial agreement with other raters, more importantly, he or she did not use the defined categories of the coding system as they were intended and did so without the researcher's knowledge—thus, the validity of the rating scheme was compromised. Due to humans' limited information processing capacities, raters frequently commit errors, especially when category, frequency, and intensity ratings are required of them. While errors in rating are not desirable, not all errors are bias because bias has to be systematic error such as that described by the halo effect.

When working clinically, dance/movement therapists need to be especially aware of how their own biases affect their movement observations. In this situation the therapist usually has access to historical and other information about the client that can bias his or her judgments of their movement behaviors, or create *observer contamination* (Borg & Gall, 1983). One way that researchers try to eliminate this type of bias in research observation is to make sure that observers are blind to information about the participants that might affect their ratings. To use Goodman's study again as an example, raters did not know which boys were with and without hyperactivity symptoms when they rated their movements. In addition, there are two other types of rater bias that need to be guarded against. One of these is the *error of leniency*, which is the tendency of a rater to rate most participants at either the high or low end of the scale used. The *error of central tendency* describes the proclivity of raters to use the middle or average of a scale for all observations (Borg & Gall, 1983). While LMA training sensitizes observers and balances their repertoire, raters' own movement preferences and biases can still influence the perceptual process. McCoubrey (1984, 1987) suggested that raters tend to either overestimate or underestimate the presence of their own personal movement preferences in observed participants. In the absence of norms, experience and comparison of profiles during training might help raters to overcome their biases and lead to better agreement among them. Unfortunately, observers can be biased even if they agree and the researcher will not know that the ratings are biased. It is even possible for rater training to be biased in a certain direction, and of course, this bias will be present in ratings that are made after training. In order to control for biases of observers, the researcher may want to compare trained observers' judgments with those of untrained observers, or judgments of raters trained in the same system but by different experts. Rater bias negatively affects validity, and thus is a serious concern.

The measurement and statistical analysis of observer agreement alone are not conclusive to support that the movement observations have been recorded accurately. The context and process of the observation and the specific conditions of the ratings always need to be considered. The quality criteria we describe below are not limited to observations; they can be applied to any kind of agreement in judgments, for example, on psychological tests or the analysis of interview data.

CRITERIA FOR SCIENTIFIC OBSERVATIONS

Validity

Validity is the degree to which an observation or instrument measures what it is supposed to measure. It is the adequacy and appropriateness of the measure for its intended application. Validity is actually more important than reliability for both research and clinical observations because while reliability is necessary, it is not sufficient for establishing the validity of observations. For example, intelligence tests can produce reliable scores for individuals across different examiners. Yet, debate in education centers around what intelligence tests actually measure (validity) because of the strong relationships of intelligence test scores to formal education, socioeconomic status, and other constructs. Ideally, intelligence test scores should measure "intelligence" and not other constructs like amount of formal education. Validity questions and issues related to DMT might be, for example, if KMP rhythms really measures physiological and psychological needs (Loman, 1995), or if indeed KMP rhythms measure some other characteristic.

Another example of validity related to DMT is represented by an investigation of the MPI that attempted to support the validity of the MPI as a measure of involuntary movement disorders (Cruz, 1995). Involuntary movement disorders are typically exhibited by patients with schizophrenia and other mental disorders and were described over 100 years ago by neurologists and psychiatrists. In Cruz's validity study, MPI data for diagnosed patients mapped to the known continuum (from absence of movement to excessive movement) of involuntary movements. The involuntary movements neurologists traditionally describe are quite noticeable compared to the subtle distinctions of the MPI. Thus the mapping of the MPI to the known continuum of involuntary movement disorder led to the conclusion that the items of the MPI may describe a finer distinction of involuntary movement disorder associated with different types of psychopathology. This one piece of information helps to make arguments about what the MPI measures. Yet, a single validity demonstration is rarely enough. There are different types of validity, as we will discuss shortly, and demonstrations of several of the different types are needed for a strong argument about the validity of an instrument or scale.

Validity is not an established or general attribute of an instrument or observation. For example, the MPI has no validity for use with individuals without severe psychiatric illnesses or children, because its use has not been tested with them. This means that in order to use the MPI with children, validity testing would need to be done first. So, validity is always associated with a demonstrated, specific use of an instrument or observation and a specific population. Since the 1950s, the American Psychological Association (APA, 1954) and the American Educational Research Association (AERA, 1955) have distinguished validity as an important element of testing standards and guidelines. There are different forms of validity, and we will discuss the major types: content, criterion, and construct validity.

Content Validity

Content validity revolves around a central question that Feder and Feder (1998, p. 56) posed in the following way, "How representative is the assessment procedure of the universe of relevant tasks and situations that have been employed?" Content validity involves carefully defining the domain to be measured and covering all important areas of this domain (Allen & Yen, 1979), and Goodman (1991) again provides an example relevant to DMT. She was interested in noting hyperactive behavior and began with a list of movement behaviors representative of that domain. Often researchers use logical judgment to determine content validity. For example, one might ask, "what does my common sense tell me about the validity of observing these characteristics?" It is possible to use expert interviews and consult empirical findings and descriptive studies to assist in this process. The degree of content validity can only be estimated, not calculated, and the methods of establishing content validity—by opinion or examination of the items to be observed—are admittedly subjective. It stands to reason then, that content validity alone is not sufficient for an observation tool. However, the process of determining content validity is very useful. Such a process entails clearly and exhaustively defining the construct or constructs that one is attempting to measure with the observation tool. A construct is an abstract idea about some characteristics or qualities individuals possess or exhibit. It cannot be directly observed, but needs to be inferred from certain directly observable behaviors that are believed to be related to the construct to certain degrees (Brunswik, 1956). For example, motor signs of anxiety may be a construct a dance/movement therapist is interested in observing, but before he or she begins observing movements that might be signs of anxiety, it is necessary to fully and completely define what the therapist or researcher means when the word anxiety is used. Definitions are likely to differ, so good researchers need to explain exactly what is meant when they use the construct, anxiety. Creating this very specific description for a construct is referred to as an *operational definition*.

Face validity is a type of content validity that is important for certain types of tests. It describes the condition of someone examining a test, and based on this examination judging that it appears to measure the relevant trait. Imagine using a movement observation scale to screen a secretarial job applicant. While the movement observation scale might actually identify a good secretary, to most people it would seem to have no relationship to performing the duties of a secretary (for example, answering phones and filing) so it would not have face validity. Face validity is more of an issue with paper and pencil tests, but our example shows that it might apply to the use of movement observations also. One way to conceptualize face validity is in terms of the face validity of DMT. When DMT first began to be practiced in institutions, treated individuals showed dramatic changes in affect and initiation during sessions that were remarkable to staff watching the sessions. On the face of it, DMT appeared an effective treatment and this phenomenon remains the same today.

Criterion Validity

Criterion validity also addresses the question of how representative the scale or targeted observations are, but for criterion validity actual data are needed. That is because it is necessary to demonstrate an empirical or data-based connection between what is observed and some other criterion of behavior measurement. Often, the researcher uses other tests that are supposed to measure the same construct or expert ratings as a criterion measure. There are two subtypes of criterion validity, concurrent and predictive. For *concurrent criterion validity* one chooses another similar measure. For example, when Judith Kestenberg examined the concurrent criterion validity of the KMP she checked whether the diagnosis derived from the KMP and Anna Freud's diagnosis from her psychoanalytic method corresponded for the same children (Kestenberg-Amighi, personal communication, October 1997). *Predictive criterion validity*, on the other hand, involves using a criterion measure of some future behavior, for example, response to treatment. To use Goodman (1991) again as an example, two of her studies examined the relationship of qualitative movement features to attention deficit hyperactivity disorder and used treatment response to medication targeting hyperactivity as the predictive criterion. Noted decreases in the observed movement features that followed beginning the medication supported that the movement features were in fact related to hyperactivity and constituted evidence for predictive criterion validity.

Establishing criterion validity requires thoughtful construction. Observational scales are rarely employed in multiples for comparison purposes due to the cost and labor factors involved when trained raters are needed. Because of this, alternative instruments may be used to measure the constructs in question to create the criterion, but the validity of these alternative instruments needs to be supported by empirical studies, and the researcher needs to make sure that all instruments measure the construct of interest as she or he has operationally defined it.

A final, technical issue that we have talked around so far is what constitutes data and how data should be treated to examine criterion validity. Each research participant needs to have a score or scores generated by the movement observation scale and a score or scores on the criterion scale, test, or measure. Depending on whether these scores are categories (yes, no), ordered categories (none, some, much), or meaningful numbers like frequency counts, the relationship between them has to be assessed using statistics that are appropriate for this purpose. Often, correlation coefficients are calculated for this purpose, but the number of individuals used in the study should be rather large. There is no absolute number that we can recommend, but as a guideline, twenty participants would be the minimum number that could be used. While an introduction to statistics is beyond the scope of this chapter, we encourage readers to consult some of the readable, conceptual treatments of statistics that are available (see for example, Kachigan, 1991; Huck & Cormier, 1996).

Construct Validity

Construct validity is essentially theory-driven because it is used to argue that the coded behavior truly assesses an individual's status on the hypothetical construct, for example, "temperament" or "anxiety." The researcher starts by defining a construct and then proposes to measure it using a movement observation scale. When he or she begins to examine construct validity, the question asked is "Now what are scores on this scale *really* related to?" The researcher has theorized about the relationship between the construct and the scale, but now it is necessary to have some actual proof of this relationship. In a formal sense, the questions for construct validity can be stated this way: How valid is the observational data for the aims and decisions the researcher wants to draw from it? Does the instrument provide the means or conditions to reach the goals for which it was created? Construct validation is a pragmatic and thorough type of validity (Allen & Yen, 1979).

There are different types of evidence that can be used to argue for construct validity. Showing that results from the use of a scale conform with theory is one type; movement characteristics measured should change or not change in a manner predicted by theory for this type of construct validity to be supported. For example, if a researcher measures movement features related to stable personality characteristics, he or she would not expect these to change over time and could measure individuals at several points in time to demonstrate the lack of change. On the other hand, if the researcher proposes that the movement features measured are related to disturbance in functioning and should change as a result of treatment, he or she might observe individuals before and after treatment and measure the amount of change as an indication of construct validity.

A third method is to demonstrate differences between groups that *should* have differences on the scale. For example, the study mentioned earlier of the MPI (Cruz, 1995) demonstrated different patterns of abnormal involuntary movements for two diagnostic groups, patients with schizophrenia spectrum disorders and those with personality disorders, who were expected to have differences. *Convergent* and *divergent* (sometimes called discriminate) validity are particularly useful in constructing demonstrations for construct validity. For *convergent validity* one shows strong relationships between the scale and other measures of the construct, while *divergent validity* involves demonstrating that the scale is not related to measures of other constructs unrelated to the one chosen. For example, if the dance/movement therapist or researcher expects a movement observation scale to measure stable personality characteristics, he or she would also expect scores on this scale not to be related to a measure of socioeconomic status.

Reliability

In its simplest form, reliability is defined as the consistency of the *scores*. We emphasize the word scores in the previous sentence because it is easy to fall into thinking of reliability as a property of a test or instrument, but in fact, it is just for a set of scores. The theory behind how one determines accuracy is actually quite interesting. Measurement theory is concerned with how the researcher determines the "goodness" of scores that result from measuring different characteristics of people. It is organized around classical test theory which some researchers also call weak true-score theory or large-sample theory (Lord & Novick, 1968). But all of these terms refer to the idea that when an individual's measurement is taken on some characteristic, the score given (called an observed score) has a relationship to a hypothetical "true" score. The relationship is that observed scores are equal to the true score plus some amount of measurement error; reliability is the estimate of how much measurement error is contained in the scores produced by a measurement procedure. This is true whenever tests are given, or even as we will discuss below, movement observations are made. Measurement error is the essence of reliability. So what is measurement error really?

Measurement error is random or unsystematic variation that can be created by a great range of things. Note that measurement error is random or unsystematic so it is not the same as *bias*. For example, if one takes a test on a day he or she is not feeling well, performance may be poor and the resulting test score may not be close to one's "true" test score. Most importantly for movement observations, measurement error can be created when two raters disagree about what they see.

Frequently one sees the terms *rater agreement* and *inter-rater reliability* used interchangeably in the literature. However, strictly speaking, measurement theory demands that these terms only be used when specific types of calculations have been employed to examine the extent of concurrence of the raters. When researchers check to see that raters agree, using percent agreement, Cohen's kappa, Kendall's tau, or even Pearson correlation coefficients (we will describe some of these in more depth presently) they should not refer to the resulting values for these measures as *inter-rater reliability* because none of them quantify measurement error, the essence of reliability. It is more correct to refer to values for these indices as evidence of *rater agreement*. One should only use the term *inter-rater reliability* to refer to a calculation that quantifies measurement error, such as the *intra-class correlation coefficient* or the *generalizability coefficient* produced by using generalizability theory.

Because of this distinction, we will use the term *inter-rater agreement* in our discussion below of percent agreement and Cohen's kappa. We will address how inter-rater agreement can be calculated, and we will introduce several ways of measuring inter-rater agreement. In addition, we will introduce a method for calculating inter-rater reliability—generalizability theory (g-theory). But first, we will finish our introduction to reliability by briefly mentioning some different methods of examining reliability when observers are not used.

A common form of reliability is *test-retest* reliability, which is used to examine the stability of an instrument or scale. Obviously the behavior or characteristic targeted by the scale should be rather stable, or this method is not appropriate. For example, when measuring teachers' reports of aggression in preschool children, test-retest reliability might appear to be low, when it is the specific behavior which is not stable. Stability of behavior needs to be carefully considered. In addition, this method involves giving the same test twice, so paper and pencil measures given a brief time apart may show similarity of scores because individuals remember the test. In our example, teachers might remember how they answered about individual children the first time and want to appear consistent in their responses.

Split-half reliability is another method in which a single instrument or scale is separated into two equivalent halves, making two scores for each individual. If the two scores are closely related, one can argue for the consistency of content sampling for the test. *Parallel-test* reliability uses two tests, A and B, with parallel constructions of similar items identical in difficulty. This method helps address the problem of individuals remembering the test. A fourth common method is *interitem consistency* as a reliability indicator of the content sampling and homogeneity of the behavior domain that is sampled by the test.

As the reader probably gathers, these forms of estimating reliability pertain to classroom and paper and pencil psychological tests. The formulas involved for calculating reliability coefficients for each of these methods relates them to true score theory. Details on these calculations are beyond the scope of this chapter, but can be found in most measurement texts including Anastasi (1988) and Allen and Yen (1979).

We described the importance of objectivity and validity previously, and pointed out the importance of reliability as an element of these criteria. However, reliability has another, very important aspect related to research, and that is the central role that reliability of measurements plays in the statistical calculations that are used to test hypotheses in research studies. The best treatment-control group study of DMT will fail to find a difference between groups if there is too much measurement error (unreliability) in the scores that are analyzed to examine the effect of the study. That happens because measurement error obscures the systematic effects of the treatments. The interested reader can use the statistics texts we mentioned for a more detailed explanation—but suffice it to say that failing to find a statistically significant effect after the work of conducting a research study is quite disheartening! For the movement observation data that is the focus here, we now look at methods of calculating rater agreement.

Inter-rater Agreement

When one uses movement observation as a form of measurement for research, it is necessary to consider inter-rater agreement as the focus of the reliability demonstration. Inter-rater agreement is defined as the degree to which different observers concur in their observations and thus implies agreement of: (a) scores; and (b) interpretations, conclusions, and diagnostic inferences made on the basis of scores. It can be established using many different methods that range from simple percent agreement, to more sophisticated and accurate calculations such as Cohen's kappa and Kendall's tau. Before entering into the types of calculations that can be used for examining inter-rater agreement, we want to briefly review the important criteria that these calculations support.

According to Graumann (1966), scientific observation is distinguished from everyday observation solely by being subject to the criterion of replicability, meaning that a different person observing the same behavior will come to the same observational result. The accuracy of the observer can be established, for example, if there is an "objective" or standard protocol that reflects by definition what the "correct" observation is. Such a protocol can be established by an expert rater. Note that when we speak of accuracy here we move into the realm of validity. Training to a criterion such as an expert rater offers a means of arguing for the validity of the observations the rater makes, but does not establish the reliability of the rater. In this case "false positives" or erroneously coded actions that have actually not taken place and "false negatives"—actions that have actually taken place but have not been coded—can be identified by comparing raters to the expert. An expert rater is not a necessity, but keeping this purpose of the expert rater in mind can help establish the validity of a movement observation scale, but does not directly impact on establishing inter-rater agreement; more is needed for that purpose.

Calculating Inter-rater Agreement

Given the importance of inter-rater agreement, how does one go about calculating it? Many of the indices that exist for this purpose follow similar principles, and depend on the way in which the scale produces information. Does the scale produce categories (yes, no), ordered categories (none, some, much), or meaningful numbers? The type of data that the scale produces determines what types of calculations can be used for inter-rater agreement.

Simple Percent Agreement

This type of calculation is particularly good for data that are categories or ordered categories, but could also be used for meaningful numbers that are summarized by the scale. For example, ratings on the MPI can be summarized over items in each of 10 categories into a single score for that category (see Davis, 1991). Simple percent agreement uses a point-by-point check of ratings, and is calculated by the following formula.

$$\% = [\text{Agreements} / (\text{Agreements} + \text{Nonagreements})] \times 100$$

In its usual form, coding is done in given time intervals so one can be sure that raters coded the exact same behavior, and each interval is judged as to whether the observers agree in their rating or not. However, other applications of percent agreement can be found in the literature. Simple percent agreement is a good heuristic for rater agreement because it is easily calculated. However, in many cases it is too undifferentiated for scientific purposes. For example, for rare events, it provides artificially increased values. Bijou and colleagues (1969, cited in Mees & Selg, 1977) suggest calculating the results for agreements and nonagreements separately for more accuracy. So, while simple percent agreement can serve as a good heuristic and can be useful for getting a quick estimate of rater agreement in the rater training phase, it can fail to take important factors into consideration, such as, agreement by chance. The next method we will discuss, Cohen's kappa, is considered a better overall index because it takes the possibility of chance agreement into consideration.

Cohen's Kappa

In clinical diagnosis, a patient may be assigned one or more out of a number of categories (depression, phobia, etc.) that do not have any hierarchy or ranking. The technical term for this type of data is *nominal* data. We will treat Cohen's kappa for nominal data more extensively than any other coefficient mentioned, because many types of data lend themselves to this coefficient. In observational studies it is possible to reach high values of rater agreement merely by chance—especially in observations with a low number of categories. In calculations of simple percent agreement the probability of reaching rater agreement by chance is not accounted for. Cohen (1960) developed a method that controlled for the chance probability of rater agreement. He suggested subtracting the agreement expected by chance from the agreement of the observation. This measure is the statistic known as *Cohen's kappa*, and we will demonstrate its calculation below.

To illustrate the calculation of kappa, imagine us (Sabine and Robyn) as two raters observing and rating a sample of dance/movement therapists on their use of space effort, direct and indirect. We observe videotapes of twenty-five individual dance/movement therapists telling a two-minute story. Our rating scheme demands that we note whether each dance/movement therapist uses primarily directness or indirectness, and we each assign a single score to rate each dance/movement therapist—0 if we saw them primarily use indirectness and 1 if we saw primarily directness. Once the raters have viewed the tapes in isolation and rated the participants by assigning a score, the data can be tabulated by entering the scores into a computer spreadsheet or even listing them out by hand with pencil and paper. The tabulated data will look like Table 4-I below. To read this table, choose the row labeled "DMT 1," which represents the scores for the first dance/movement therapist in the sample, and by reading across the row it is possible to see that Robyn and Sabine both rated this dance/movement therapist as using primarily direct space effort (both gave a "1" for direct). So the dance/movement therapist participants make up the rows of the table and the dance/movement therapists' identification numbers and ratings are in the three columns.

Next, it is necessary to summarize the data across all the dance/movement therapists to prepare for calculating Cohen's kappa, and this is done by counting the number of agreements and disagreements for each category. Using the data in Table 4-I, it is possible to see that we agreed on direct four times and indirect twenty times (and we had one disagreement). Table 4-II shows the setup used to summarize the data (called a crosstabulation) on agreements and disagreements to prepare to calculate Cohen's kappa for the case of two observers using two categories for rating.

To calculate Cohen's kappa with the paper-and-pencil method we use a formula below simplified to facilitate easy calculation (Cohen, 1960).

Table 4-I   OBSERVATION DATA EXAMPLE

DMT#	ROBYN	SABINE
1	1.00	1.00
2	.00	.00
3	.00	.00
4	.00	.00
5	.00	.00
6	.00	.00
7	.00	.00
8	.00	.00
9	.00	1.00
10	.00	.00
11	.00	.00
12	.00	.00
13	.00	.00
14	.00	.00
15	.00	.00
16	.00	.00
17	.00	.00
18	1.00	1.00
19	.00	.00
20	.00	.00
21	.00	.00
22	1.00	1.00
23	1.00	1.00
24	.00	.00
25	.00	.00

Note: 1=Direct, 0=Indirect

Table 4-II   COUNTS SUMMARIZING OBSERVATIONS BY
TWO RATERS USING TWO CATEGORIES

Robyn	Sabine		
	Indirect	Direct	Total
Indirect	20	1	21
Direct	0	4	4
Total	20	5	25

$$\text{kappa} = (f_{\text{observed}} - f_{\text{chance}}) / (N - f_{\text{chance}})$$

Where f_{observed} = frequency of units on which judges agreed,
f_{chance} = frequency of agreement expected by chance, and
N = total number of units

It is easy to find the frequency of units on which judges agreed from Table 4-II. They agreed twenty dance/movement therapists were indirect and four were direct, so f_{observed} = 24. Finding the frequency of agreements by chance is also easy, but we have to use the numbers labeled "total" in Table 4-II. For chance agreements on indirect multiply the numbers labeled *total* that are directly below and across from the agreements on indirect (20 and 21) and divide by the total number of dance/movement therapists (25). For chance agreements on direct use the numbers labeled *total* that are directly opposite and below the number of agreements on direct (5 and 4) and again divide by the total number of therapists rated. Our actual calculations are:

$$f_o = 24$$

$$f_c = [(20 \times 21)/25] + [(4 \times 5)/25]$$
$$= 16.8 + 0.8$$
$$= 17.6$$

$$\text{kappa} = (f_o - f_c) / (N - f_c)$$

$$\text{kappa} = (24 - 17.6) / (25 - 17.6)$$
$$= 6.4 / 7.4$$
$$= .865$$

Values of kappa range from 0.0 to 1.0 (perfect agreement), and obviously the closer the value of kappa is to 1, the better the agreement. To compare the value of kappa obtained in the example to the value of percent agreement, percent agreement can be calculated for the data. The formula and calculation are:

$$\% = [\text{Agreements} / (\text{Agreements} + \text{Disagreements})] \times 100$$

$$= 24/(24 + 1) \times 100$$
$$= 24/25 \times 100$$
$$= .96 \times 100$$
$$= 96\% \text{ agreement}$$

While the values of kappa and percent agreement cannot be directly compared because they are in different metrics, remember that by using kappa agreement by chance has been taken into consideration and thus produces a more defendable index of rater agreement. In this case, because 80 percent of the dance/movement therapists were judged indirect (20/25), chance agreement for indirect was a little more than 64 percent (16/25 = .64). Knowing that our agreement was good even when this amount of chance agreement was possible is even more impressive.

Researchers can use statistical software programs like SPSS to calculate Cohen's kappa. To analyze the data in our example with SPSS, we entered the data exactly as shown in Table 4-I above. Then, using SPSS for Windows, we selected Analyze, then Descriptives, and Crosstabs from the pull-down menus. This produces access to a window where we entered the variables we wanted to compare. We entered the variable with one rater's ratings in the box for "column" and the variable representing the other rater's ratings in the box for "rows." Finally we selected the Statistics button and checked "kappa" and then selected "ok." The analysis appears in the output window. For the analysis of the example data, the SPSS output results are below in Figure 4-1. Note that the value of kappa (.865) is the same as the value obtained when it was calculated by hand.

Interpretation of kappa is the amount of agreement better than chance agreement. This is because chance agreement has been removed from the kappa coefficient during calculation. While there are no hard and fast rules

Robyn * Sabine Crosstabulation

			Sabine		
			Indirect	*Direct*	*Total*
Robyn	Indirect	Count	20	1	21
		Expected Count	16.8	4.2	21.0
	Direct	Count	0	4	4
		Expected Count	3.2	.8	4.0
Total		Count	20	5	25
		Expected Count	20.0	5.0	25.0

Symmetric Measures

		Value	*Asymp. Std. Error^a*	*Approvx. T^b*	*Approx. Sign.*
Measure of Agreement	Kappa	.865	.131	4.364	.000
N of Valid Cases		25			

Key: ^{a}Not assuming the null hypothesis.
^{b}Using the asymptotic standard error assuming the null hypothesis.

Figure 4-1   Output From SPSS for Calculating Cohen's Kappa for Example Data

Table 4-III   CRITERIA FOR THE INTERPRETATION
OF KAPPA VALUES BY LANDIS & KOCH (1977)

Kappa	*Interpretation*
.00–.20	Slight
.21–40	Fair
.41–.60	Moderate
.61–.80	Substantial
> .80	Almost Perfect

for what constitutes a "good" or "poor" value of kappa, Landis & Koch (1977) provided some criteria for the interpretation of kappa (see Table 4-III).

The value of kappa for our example falls in the "almost perfect" range. If the dance/movement therapists had been rated on other characteristics, it would be possible to compute kappa for those characteristics also. For data where scores are ordered (for example, none, some, a little), there is a weighted kappa coefficient (Cohen, 1968). It can be applied, for example, in ratings of whether a person displays "no evidence," "slight evidence," or "strong evidence" of the movement characteristic rated.

In some situations, the maximum value of kappa is not 1.0 but less than 1.0. For example if the characteristic observed is rather rare, this causes the kappa value to be affected. It can be helpful to calculate kappa$_{max}$ to know the maximum value possible. Dividing the obtained kappa value by kappa$_{max}$ tells us how much of the allowable agreement is present (see Cohen, 1960, for the formula).

Sometimes observational ratings produce data that are meaningful numbers such as frequencies of occurrence. For this type of *interval* data there are other options. One option, the *intraclass correlation coefficient* (ICC; Ebel, 1951), can also be used with data that are ordered or *ordinal* such as Likert-scale ratings of efforts (for example, rating how someone uses lightness on a scale from 1 to 4). The ICC is calculated by partitioning variance in the scores using analysis of variance. The next method we will discuss is an extension of the ICC that is more useful because it allows examination of raters, items, and their interactions at the same time. This method is called generalizability theory and can be helpful in rater training and for examining rater behavior.

Generalizability Theory

Cronbach, Gleser, Nanda, and Rajaratnam (1972) described generalizability theory as a technique that provides a broader frame than the classical reliability concepts for assessing the quality of observational data. Generalizability theory (g-theory) provides estimates of how much variability in a set of scores or ratings can be attributed to different sources. For example, variability can be created by the participants, the raters, and the items of the scale. In addition, those three components can interact and g-theory allows the examination of those interactions as well. Why is this important? Well, one wants to make sure that raters are functioning as knowledgably as possible, so it might be of interest to know if some raters "see" more of certain behaviors described by the scale items than others. One of the benefits of using g-theory is that it is possible to have more than two raters, a situation that is not easily handled with kappa or other agreement indicators (but see Fleiss, 1971). Another benefit is that g-theory allows the calculation of a generalizability coefficient that is a true reliability coefficient so it includes quantification of measurement error.

To be more specific, the effects captured in each component of a g-theory design can be interpreted according to guidelines established by Shavelson and Webb (1991). If the design has participants, raters, and items, the *participants* component calculated with g-theory indicates how participants differed from one another in their movement behavior. The *raters* component shows the extent to which some raters "saw" more movement behaviors than others. The *items* component reveals if the average level of some movement behavior items was higher than others. The *participants by raters* interaction indicates if the relative standing of participants' movement behavior changed from rater to rater; that some participants and raters in combination produced a unique result. The *raters by items* interaction reveals inconsistencies of raters' average ratings from item to item, for example, whether a rater liberally noted one item over all subjects but not the next item. The *participants by items* interaction can show inconsistency of relative standing of participants from item to item. For example, a participant might show high frequency on one item but not on other items. Finally, the *residual* component reflects variance from the three-way interaction of participants, items, and raters that cannot be separated from unmeasured or unspecified sources of error variance. With g-theory one can directly compare the proportions of variance due to all of the above components and their interactions. For example, when raters are in agreement, the proportion of variance accounted for by raters and other components representing interactions with raters (i.e., raters × items, raters × participants) should be small relative to components that do not include raters. A complete example of using g-theory can be found in Koch, Cruz, and Goodill (2002). We will summarize this study briefly below.

Koch, Cruz, and Goodill (2002) studied the rating behavior of five student raters who had been trained in the KMP. Their training took place in a uniform manner and their observations were made using uniformly videotaped participants from a community dance group. The study used a g-theory design for analysis with the components described above, participants, raters, items, and their interactions. A summary of the g-theory results for the ratings of the KMP tension-flow rhythms is displayed in Table 4-IV.

Table 4-IV   VARIANCE COMPONENT ESTIMATES FOR TENSION-FLOW RHYTHMS
(KOCH, CRUZ, & GOODILL, 2002)

Source	Percent of Total Variance
Participants(P)	0.0
Raters(R)	0.0
Items(I)	34.1
PxR	0.0
PxI	13.2
RxI	28.0
PxRxI, e	24.8

Note: percentages do not sum to 100 due to rounding error

Analysis = Tension-flow rhythms – 10 items

PxRxI,e = Residual variance

This analysis of the ten tension-flow rhythms found that the sum of the individual components related to raters (raters, raters by participants, and raters by items) accounted for 28 percent of the total variance, but the *raters × items* interaction accounted for all of the variance associated with raters. Other large components were items (34.1%), the three-way interaction and error or the *residual* (24.8%), and the *participants × items* interaction (13.2%). The large *rater by item* interaction term indicated inconsistencies in raters' stringency from one item to another. This lack of rater consistency with items was not so surprising for novice raters given the complexity of the instrument—and especially the complexity of the rhythms ratings—but this was only detected with certainty by using g-theory.

SUMMARY

In this brief treatment of validity and reliability with specific application to movement observations, we have presented introductions to the issues that affect the scientific quality of observations. The discussion of validity and reliability and the examples of three methods of examining rater agreement were intended to give the reader a working understanding that can be applied and extended to both research and clinical practice. There are many other ways to calculate rater agreement, but we described methods that we think are of major relevance and practical applicability in observational studies. We presented a method based on simplicity (percent agreement), one that incorporates chance agreement (Cohen's kappa), and one that can be used to produce information about both the items and the raters, and how raters use items (g-theory). This hierarchy of techniques also addressed different types of data (nominal, ordinal, and interval), including different numbers of raters, and is meant to show the options that are available.

There are some remaining issues that we would like to mention. Few of the observational systems used in DMT have established norms based on large samples of individuals. This means that they cannot be used to compare individuals to larger groups of the population as it is possible, for example, to compare a child's motor development to that of other children using the Bayley Scales of Infant Development (Bayley, 1993). However, such types of comparisons might be available in the future for the KMP. K. Mark Sossin (2003) is working to establish frequency norms of KMP observations for children at different developmental stages, and while this is a task of great proportion, these norms may be available to dance/movement therapists in the near future.

There are also developments in using emerging technologies to measure movement and changes in movement. Some computer software can be used to organize and analyze movement features, for example The Observer (Noldus Information Technology, 2003), THEME (Magnusson, 2000), and Media Tagger (Brugman & Kita, 1995). While using such technology will enhance reliability and make validity studies more feasible and economical, some of this software is still quite expensive and beyond the means of unfunded researchers. Some attempts at digitalizing measurement of KMP tension-flow rhythms and attributes are in process at the Hebrew University of Jerusalem, Israel (Lotan & Yirmiya, 2002). These types of changes will create new challenges for research and theory development over the next several years.

Validity and reliability of measures, and movement observations in particular, are important considerations in both research and clinical practice. Regardless of the research methods that are used, the researcher needs to substantiate that observations are valid and reliable. This is as true for research that uses narrative or qualitative methods as it is for quantitative methods. We also want to stress the importance of clinicians formalizing their movement observations through attention to some of the ideas we have discussed in this chapter. While the discipline of systematically observing and noting changes in clients' movements and movement patterns seems a large and time consuming undertaking, this type of recording can be extremely useful documentation that improves clinical practice and supports arguments for the medical necessity of treatment. All clients insured by public or private organizations must meet the organization's definitions of medical necessity to receive treatment. Documentation of changes in movement can be used to support the success of dance/movement therapy treatment or the need to remain in treatment. We suggest that clinicians train and regularly update their training in the system of movement observation they find most useful to their population and work setting. Refreshing training directly addresses reliability and awareness of rater biases that affect the reliability of ratings. We hope that DMT researchers and clinicians will focus on the issues of validity and reliability of movement observations in an effort to move the profession forward.

Authors' Note. We thank Darrell L. Sabers, Ph.D., Professor and Head, Department of Educational Psychology, The University of Arizona, for his useful critique of this chapter.

REFERENCES

Allen, M. J., & Yen, W. M. (1979). *Introduction to measurement theory.* Monterey, CA: Brooks/Cole.

Amelang, M., & Zielinski, W. (1997). *Psychologische Diagnostik und Intervention* [Psychological Diagnostics and Intervention]. Heidelberg: Springer.

American Educational Research Association & National Council on Measurements Used in Education. (1955). *Technical recommendations for achievement tests.* Washington, DC: National Education Association.

American Psychological Association. (1954). Technical recommendations for psychological tests and diagnostic techniques. *Psychological Bulletin, 51*(2, Pt. 2).

Anastasi, A. (1988). *Psychological testing* (6th ed.). New York: Macmillan.

Bayley, N. (1993). *Bayley Scales of Infant Development* (2nd ed.). San Antonio, TX: Psychological Corporation.

Berrol, C. F., & Katz, S. S. (1990, 1993). *The Functional Assessment of Movement and Perception* (Unpublished Assessment).

Berrol, C. F., Ooi, W. L., & Katz, S. S. (1997). Dance/movement therapy with older adults who have sustained neurological insult: A demonstration project. *American Journal of Dance Therapy, 19,* 135–154.

Borg, W. R., & Gall, M. D. (1983). *Educational research: An introduction* (4th ed.). New York: Longman.

Brugman, H., & Kita, S. (1995). Impact of digital video technology on transcription: a case of spontaneous gesture transcription. *Ars Semiotica, 18,* 95–112.

Brunswik, E. (1956). *Perception and the representative design of psychological experiments.* Berkeley, CA: University of California Press.

Cohen, J. (1960). A coefficient of agreement for nominal scales. *Educational and Psychological Measurement, 20,* 37-46.

Cohen, J. (1968). Weighted kappa: nominal scale agreement with provision for scaled disagreement or partial credit. *Psychological Bulletin, 70,* 213-220.

Cronbach, L. J., Gleser, J. C., Nanda, H., & Rajaratnam, N. (1972). *The dependability of behavioral measurements: Theory of generalizability of scores and profiles.* New York: Wiley.

Cruz, R. F. (1995). An empirical investigation of the Movement Psychodiagnostic Inventory (Doctoral dissertation, The University of Arizona). *Dissertation Abstracts International (2B), (UMI No.AAM962042257).*

Davis, M. (1987). Steps to achieving observer agreement: The LIMS reliability project. *Movement Studies, 2,* 7–19.

Davis, M. (1991). *Guide to movement analysis methods part 2: Movement Psychodiagnostic Inventory.* (Unpublished manual; available from Martha Davis, 1 West 85th Street, New York, NY 10024).

Ebel, R. L. (1951). Estimation of the reliability of ratings. *Psychometrika, 16,* 407–424.

Feder, B., & Feder, E. (1998). *The art and science of evaluation in the arts therapies: How do you know what's working?* Springfield, IL: Charles C Thomas.

Fleiss, J. L. (1971). Measuring nominal scale agreement among many raters. *Psychological Bulletin, 76,* 378–382.

Gergen, K. J. (1985). The social constructionist movement in modern psychology. *American Psychologist, 40,* 266–275.

Goodman, L. S. (1991). Movement behavior of hyperactive children: A qualitative analysis. *American Journal of Dance Therapy, 13*, 19–31.

Graumann, C. F. (1966). Grundzüge der Verhaltensbeobachtung [An outline of behavioral observation]. In Hans Hörmann (Ed.), *Aussagemöglichkeiten psychologischer Diagnostik* [Possibilities of psycho-diagnosis]. Göttingen: Hogrefe.

Huck, S. W., & Cormier, W. H. (1996). *Reading statistics and research* (2nd ed.). New York: Harper Collins.

Kachigan, S. K. (1991). *Multivariate statistical analysis: A conceptual introduction* (2nd ed.). New York: Radius.

Kestenberg, J. (1975). *Children and parents: Psychoanalytic studies in development.* Northvale, NJ: Jason Aronson.

Koch, S. C., Cruz, R. F., & Goodill, S. (2002). The Kestenberg Movement Profile: Performance of novice raters. *American Journal of Dance Therapy, 23*, 71–87.

Koffka, K. (1935). *Principles of gestalt psychology.* London: Routledge.

Köhler, W. (1924/33). *Die physischen Gestalten in Ruhe und im stationären Zustand.* [The physical gestalt in stillness and in stationary state]. Erlangen: Verlage der Philosophischen Akademie.

Laban, R. (1980). *The mastery of movement.* London: MacDonald & Evans.

Laban, R., & Lawrence, F. C. (1947/74). *Effort: Economy in body movement* (2nd ed.). Boston: Plays.

Landis, J. R., & Koch, G. G. (1977). The measurement of observer agreement for categorical data. *Biometrics, 33*, 159–174.

Loman, S. (1995). *Training manual for the Kestenberg Movement Profile.* Keene, NH: Antioch New England Graduate School.

Lord, F. M., & Novick, M. R. (1968). *Statistical theories of mental test scores.* Reading, MA: Addison-Wesley.

Lotan, N., & Yirmiya, N. (2002). Body movement, presence of parents and the process of falling asleep in toddlers. *International Journal of Behavioral Development, 26*(1), 81–88.

Magnusson, M. S. (2000). Discovering hidden time patterns in behavior: T-patterns and their detection. *Behavior Research Methods: Instruments & Computers, 32*, 93–110.

McCoubrey, C. (1984). *Effort observation in movement research: An interobserver reliability study.* Unpublished masters thesis. Philadelphia: Hahnemann University.

McCoubrey, C. (1987). Intersubjectivity versus objectivity: Implications for effort observations and training. *Movement Studies, 2*, 3–6.

Mees, U., & Selg, H. (1977). *Verhaltensbeobachtung und Verhaltensmodifikation* [Behavior observation and modification]. Stuttgart: Klett.

Noldus Information Technology. (2003). The Observer (Version 5.0) [Computer software]. The Netherlands: NIT.

Saal, F. E., Downey, R. G., & Lahey, M. A. (1980). Rating the ratings: Assessing the psychometric quality of rating data. *Psychological Bulletin, 88*, 413–428.

Shavelson, R. J., & Webb, N. M. (1991). *Generalizability theory: A primer.* Newbury Park, CA: Sage.

Sossin, K. M. (2003, October). Recent statistical and normative findings regarding the KMP: Implications for theory and application. *Proceedings of the American Dance Therapy Association 37th Annual Conference*, Burlington, VT.

Wallbott, H. (1982). Audiovisual recording: Procedures, equipment, and troubleshooting. In K. Scherer & P. Ekman (Eds.), *Handbook of methods in nonverbal behavior research* (pp. 542–579). Cambridge, MA: Cambridge University Press.

Chapter 5

THE CASE STUDY

HARRIS CHAIKLIN AND SHARON CHAIKLIN

INTRODUCTION

Research creates new understanding by building on what exists. It involves risk, self-reliance, and responsibility, and is a venture into uncertainty. Being able to tolerate uncertainty is a prime requirement for the creativity which research and practice require. The case study method was a crucial research element in creating modern science (Bernard, 1949; Cohen & Nagel, 1934; Mill, 1988). It is an essential clinical research and practice tool (Charlton & Walston, 1998; Galliher, 2002; Gilgun, 1994). Hammersley and Gomm (2000) say, "In one sense all research is case study: there is always some unit, or set of units, in relation to which data are collected and/or analyzed" (p. 2).

Research has had difficulty being accepted as a necessary part of a practitioner's repertoire. Some practitioners see it as alien and reject science as an obligatory element in practice (Higgens, 2001), while some contend that practice research is intrusive and exploits patients. Practitioners tend to honor research in the breach. Most of them say it is important, but their education and practice settings do little to create conditions that demonstrate the close relationship between practice skill and research skill (Higgens, 2001).

This chapter is concerned with doing case study research in dance therapy. We examine the nature of clinical science, clinical theory, and how case studies can be scientific. We then go on to define case study, the case, and review the strengths and weaknesses of the method. This is followed by an outline for conducting a study, an illustration, and a conclusion.

Clinical Science

Even if they do not think of themselves as clinical scientists, every practitioner is doing case study research (Edwards, 1999; Herreid & Schiller, 1999). Research thinking and practice thinking are identical. Holt (1961) calls clinical judgment a "disciplined inquiry" (p. 289). Erikson reflects this when he characterizes practice as research and says that treatment proceeds "as subsequent appointments become part of a developing case which step for step verifies or contradicts whatever predictions had been made and put to test earlier" (Erikson, 1959, pp. 74–75). Any practitioner who treats individuals must follow a similar procedure (Bruch, 1974; Kassier, 1983). There is an old saying that "Technique is a dancer's freedom." Dance therapists and researchers must master a discipline before they are free to be creative in their endeavors (Chaiklin, 1968, 1997).

The differences between the case study as practice and the case study as research lie more in intent than in behavior. What differentiates the two activities is what is done with the record of practice. In the former case nothing, and in the latter case it is conceptualized and written up for publication. Practitioners who see the potential for clinical research with every person they work with may make their recording more systematic or adapt brief standardized instruments that will give them better control over how they record practice and a greater ability to compare cases (Zabora et al., 2001). When practice is presented this way it eases communication with other professionals and increases the acceptance of dance therapy as a treatment modality.

Simple instruments such as the Hopkins 90 symptom checklist, which has been shortened to an 18-item Brief Symptom Inventory, make for effective practice monitoring and have utility as research instruments (Derogatis, 1977; Stefanek, Derogartis, & Shaw, 1993). The Brief Symptom Inventory takes four minutes to administer and yields scores on depression, anxiety, somatization, and general distress.

Clinical Theory

At its core a theory is a way of looking at the world, the basis for making an interpretation. When clinicians, whether doing practice or research, are not guided by theory, they tend to have too much rather than too little information about the people with whom they work. This contributes to a lack of the necessary publication for building the profession because the data, "due to its bulk, is unwieldy and, if written up in undigested form, unreadable" (Freud, 1971, p. ix).

The theory which guides clinicians' work is often not clear to the average practitioner. Often they deny using a theory or say they are eclectic. In the first instance they forget that if they interpret behavior they are using a theory and in the second instance they do not realize that to be eclectic they must have mastery of many theories so they know which part to select to make up their eclecticism. Sometimes the theory they espouse is not the one they use (Argyris & Schön, 1974). Gottman and Leiblum (1974) say, "We believe that one of the greatest sources of worry to the novice therapist is the absence of a meaningful conceptual framework" (p. 1). This hampers both practice and research (Smitskamp, 1995).

The clinical researcher and the clinician need confidence in the judgments they form on the basis of clinical observations (Becker, 1958). Without this, it is impossible to either do clinical research or to demonstrate practice competence (McCall & Simmons, 1969; Riley & Nelson, 1974; Yin, 1989). There is reasonable evidence that dance therapy is effective, but work must be continued to solidify the scientific base of the profession (Berrol, 2000; Chaiklin, 1968, 1997; Cruz & Sabers, 1998; Ritter & Low, 1996).

One of the secondary gains which come from routinely treating practice as case study research is that the practitioner gains skill in the necessary task of connecting research findings to practice (Proctor, 2001). This is not an easy task since most practice settings are not organized to encourage thinking in research terms (Johnson, 1997).

Case Study and Science

Misunderstanding the nature of science has hindered accepting the case study as a research tool. Charlton and Walston (1998) say that "Case studies have acquired an unmerited reputation as being anecdotal, unscientific and intrinsically inferior to group studies. The subsequent disregard of individual patients as the subject of investigation has led to the neglect of an extremely useful, indeed essential, clinical research method" (p. 147).

A scientific report advances propositions and "tests them against experience with observation and experiment" (Popper, 1965, p. 27). To have doubts about the role of science and research in practice is unfortunate for it hinders seeing that the practitioner who is also a skilled researcher has an opportunity to include the patient as an equal participant in an exciting endeavor (Schön, 1983). The scientific method does not tell one what problem to study or control what happens to the results when they are published. The scientific method is a widely shared set of procedures for generating knowledge that others will accept. Understanding the basics of the scientific method includes knowing that the controlled randomized experiment is not the only acceptable research endeavor.

Case studies have made landmark and enduring contributions to social science and clinical practice. To cite only a couple of examples, the Lynds' examination of *Middletown* not only endures but has helped spawn many community studies (Lynd & Lynd, 1929). Baruch's (1952) *One Little Boy* is a work that clinicians still refer to for theoretical insights and treatment suggestions. These case studies are scientific because they are "reproducible, predictive and can be adapted to useful human endeavors" (Hall, 2002, p. 14). This stands as a pretty good definition of a clinician's responsibilities.

WHAT IS A CASE STUDY?

While there are many definitions of case study, they all have some common features. One general definition states that it is "a detailed examination of an event (or series of related events) which the analyst believes exhibits (or exhibit) the operation of some identified theoretical principle" (Mitchell, 2000, p.170). This defines the case study from the observer's point of view.

The clinical researcher should also take the client's point of view into account. Behavior does not speak for itself. It is capable of many interpretations. Each of the available interpretations represents a theory of that behavior. If a theory is not explicitly stated it can often be implied by knowing the standpoint from which the interpretation is made. A person who uses his cell phone in a theater may say "I am standing up for the principle of free speech." His friend may call him "obstinate." A therapist might cite this as an example of neurotic behavior and in some places the law would make it illegal (Merton, 1957). Each of these interpretations of behavior depends on the theoretical perspective used. When a researcher undertakes a case study it is not only necessary to be aware of the basis for interpreting data, but also of the perspective used in interpreting that data.

What Is a Case?

As with defining a case study there is no definitive solution to defining a "case." The study scope can cover a continuum that starts with an individual and ends with a community or larger entity (Axline, 1964; *Manpower and Training for Corrections*, 1964, 1966). It is rare that an original definition is created. One chooses from the range of acceptable definitions that are in use (Ragin & Becker, 1992). One technical definition is that a case is "a phenomenon for which we report and interpret only a single measure of any pertinent variable" (Eckstein, 2000, p. 124). Mitchell (2000) says that a case is the social situation in which the case study research is done (p. 170).

Strengths and Weaknesses of Case Study Research

The case study method is no better or worse than any other scientific method. Even the vaunted controlled experiment cannot guarantee that its results are definitive (Campbell, 1988). For example, controlled medical studies often use placebos. Many people figure out who is getting the placebo and others improve because of belief in the drug or procedure (Fisher & Greenberg, 1997; Shapiro & Shapiro, 1997).

The case study is the method of choice for studying on-going life situations (Tuckett, 1999). Its greatest strength is in managing multiple factors (Gomm, Hammersley, & Foster, 2000). This richness allows a focus on understanding the situation. No other research method allows simultaneously seeing the whole and the parts or moving the parts around to create different combinations. For example, a dance/movement therapist doing clinical diagnosis by assessing movement can report an overall diagnostic impression and the specific movement characteristics that went into making that diagnosis. During the diagnostic process different movement interventions can be tried as the therapist moves toward forming an estimate. This ability makes doing a case study an "insight-stimulating" experience (Jahoda, Deutsch, & Cook, 1951, p. 42).

Case studies are not usually given credit for their usefulness in helping practitioners make clinical and policy decisions (Innes, Greenfield, & Greenfield, 2000; Marshall, 1999). It is a powerful way to communicate and to help the public understand therapeutic ideas (Fonagy & Moran, 1993).

Another strength is that equal weight can be given to findings which do not support the hypothesis (Charlton & Walston, 1998). For example, in making clinical diagnoses it is easy to fall into a pattern where diagnostic indicators are used rigidly. One criterion for major depression is having a depressed mood most of the day. There are cases of "masked depression" where this feature is not present. In all research there are data that do not fit expectations. These are called discrepant data or deviant cases. The case study is ideally suited to examine exceptions to what is considered the general rule. The practitioner alert to these possibilities will often find a path to new ideas and discoveries.

The weaknesses in case study research are related to misdiagnosis, inappropriate case selection, dependence on memory, and the same methodological difficulties that occur with any attempt to measure and record behavior (Charlton & Walston, 1998). These limitations are surmountable. Spence (1993), for example, suggests a way for therapists to deal with dependence on memory by tape recording exact statements and comments on the therapeutic interchange.

DOING THE STUDY

Study Goals: What Is the Problem?

Where do ideas come from? Some use phrases such as "critical common sense," "felt discomfort," and "the irritation of doubt" to describe the sense of being bothered enough by something to want to find out about it (Fisch, 1986; Skagestad, 1981). Without this divine exasperation, research is an onerous task. To begin doing research it is necessary to want to find out about something. The researcher must own the issue. When this is done the researcher finds that advisors, consultants, and friends can be extremely helpful because the researcher knows what advice fits into the project and what doesn't.

Writing the problem statement commences the research (Reynolds, 1971). This translates that sense of being curious about something into a concrete procedure. It also involves making a value judgment. A problem is picked over other possible choices. This is a judgment and not a bias. A judgment is a choice among available options. The researcher must spell this out and defend it in making a proposal or grant application.

An initial problem statement should be in the form of a declarative sentence or a question. "I want to know if dance therapy can effect change in the movement patterns of a person with bulimia." Statements longer than this usually are too complex. They introduce an information overload both for the person who states the problem and the listener who tries to understand what the question is about.

Approaches to Case Study Research

There are two approaches to doing the case study. One is inductive and the other is deductive. Inductive studies don't have formulated hypotheses, but work with broad statements of aims. In the example being used here a dance therapist might say, "I am working with someone who has bulimia and I would like to find out if dance therapy affects their movement patterns." It is easy to undertake such a study but hard to finish it. There are few indicators of what data to collect so it is easy to collect more than is needed. In order to interpret the data many theories have to be known to find the one that fits the data best (Chaiklin, 1975; Ruddock, 1972). The findings are after the fact (ex post facto) and for them to be accepted, the study must be repeated by proceeding deductively.

A deductive study is theory based. The concepts in the hypothesis direct the researcher toward the data that needs to be collected and how it is to be interpreted (Good & Scates, 1954; Yin, 1989). Techniques only manipulate the hypotheses to test the theory being used (Kaplan, 1964). The researcher can visualize what the data presentation will look like at the time of formulating the proposal.

A theory-based statement of the initial question could be: "I want to find out if using the Chace concept of shared rhythms in dance therapy will change the movement patterns of a person with bulimia, as specified by Stark, Aronow, & McGeehan" (Stark, Aronow, & McGeehan, 1989; Sandel, Chaiklin, & Lohn, 1993). The researcher can specify the intervention technique to be used and the basis for the categories to be used in observing the movement data.

When a theory-based research question is formulated the researcher has an idea of how to proceed in answering the question. A non-theory-based question involves the researcher in time consuming trial and error. There is a difference between presenting a case study where the intervention is explicitly described in terms of the Chace technique of shared rhythms and one where the research can only describe the intervention in terms that are unique to the therapist. This limits the ability to communicate ideas to others.

If there is not a lot of time to do a study it is best to think of developing a design where data are collected only once. In any study which proposes to examine a change in behavior, time becomes a variable and data must be collected at least twice. This is a particularly significant consideration for those who want to do clinical case studies. Change takes time. It is tempting for clinicians to propose studies that reflect the effects of intervention. In doing so they should make careful estimates of the time it takes to achieve the change. A common error is seen in studies that postulate that a limited number of group sessions will help people achieve major changes in their character structure, such as achieving identity. It takes several years before one knows whether such interventions help someone achieve an identity (Erikson, 1968, 1975).

The idea has primacy over methods. There is always a way to research a good idea, but the best techniques will never rescue a bad idea. In the example above the problem statement dealt with the question of whether dance therapy could help change the movement patterns of a bulimic. With an accurate diagnosis from the *Diagnostic and Statistical Manual of Mental Disorders IV* (DSM-IV; American Psychiatric Association, 1994), and a way to reflect movement patterns and to record the dance therapy interventions, there is enough information to do an excellent descriptive case study. The optimal mind set in doing research is to work on only one part of the project at a time while keeping the whole endeavor in mind.

The Hypothesis

An hypothesis is a statement of relationship between concepts. When a research question is stated in inductive terms no hypothesis is possible. It would have to be formulated after the study. In the theory-based question posed earlier, the hypothesis was implicit. Changing the initial problem statement into an hypothesis, it becomes, "There is a relationship between using Chace's shared rhythms in dance therapy and change in the movement patterns of a person with bulimia, as specified by Stark, Aronow, & McGeehan (1989)." This hypothesis is short, clear, and understandable. Hypotheses should not have more than two or three concepts. Otherwise the argument becomes too complex to report on easily.

There are two concepts in this hypothesis: "shared rhythms" and "movement pattern." There is a third, bulimia, but this is considered a defining condition of the study and is established before it begins. This is done by comparing behavior to the *DSM-IV* (1994) criteria (coded 307.51 for bulimia). Among these criteria are an excessive emphasis on body shape and weight, problems with self-esteem, and many depressive and anxiety symptoms. The most prominent symptom is binge eating at least twice a week for three months followed by some attempt to deal with the excessive intake by purging (*DSM-IV*, 1994).

Chace worked from a psychoanalytic base which emphasized Harry Stack Sullivan's interpersonal methods, Frieda Fromm-Reichamann's use of interpersonal and objects relations theory, Jarl Dyrud's ability to integrate psychoanalytic treatment with other treatment techniques, and Jacob L. Moreno's psychodrama. She emphasized interaction and working with the healthy parts of the person. Siegel said that "Chace's great contribution consisted to a large extent in making the abstract formulations of psychoanalysis and developmental psychology concretely accessible in her creation of dance therapy" (Siegel, 1993, p. 170).

In her theoretical integration Chace emphasized four things, body action, symbolism, relationship in therapeutic movement, and rhythmic activity (Chaiklin & Schmais, 1993). Each of these elements is broken down into a set of specific goals whose presence or absence can be observed. The concept of shared rhythms is derived from these four elements.

Here the hypothesis is stated as an exploratory hypothesis: that is, the type and direction of the change is not predicted. It is usually better to use this form since seldom is enough known to make firm predictions. It is also best to test only one or two hypotheses. To attempt to test too many hypotheses will swamp a project.

One thing should be noted about clinical intervention hypotheses. They always have a causal element in that a therapist does not intervene unless they expect change. In this instance the exploratory element is retained in that the direction of change is not predicted, and while a positive outcome is hoped for, it is not stated as a formal goal of the research (also see Chapter 3 in this volume for more discussion of hypotheses).

Such a study is efficient since the question to be answered is whether the data conform to the hypothesis (Nagel, 1961). In clinical practice a hypothesis is considered accepted if behavior matches the prediction (Erikson, 1959; Meehl, 1954). Whether it does or doesn't, the therapist makes a new hypothesis before proceeding (Erikson, 1959). That is the nature of therapy. When an intervention works the therapist has to formulate an approach for working with the next stage of the problem. When it doesn't work the therapist must develop a new intervention hypothesis. It is only by being aware of the basis of his or her treatment techniques that a therapist can account for the outcome of treatment in a way that other professionals will accept.

Operationally Define Key Concepts

An operational definition is the procedure by which key concepts are made evident (Feigl, 1945). A concept is an idea that sums up a class of facts. Concepts without an empirical referent are not useful for research. It is often possible to find a measure in studies used in the review of literature.

A concept must have a minimum of two categories which are logical, mutually exclusive, exhaustive, and theoretically relevant. When concepts are operationally defined, the facts that allow placing data in a category of the concept are specified. Categories can be collapsed but they can't be expanded, so it is a safety measure to start with more categories than one ends up with. For example, "shared rhythms" has categories such as "moving together" and "moving in synchrony." To be useful in research and practice these labels must be further subdivided or noted as "present," "absent," or for example, rated from "1-10." Numerical categories can then be collapsed into "Hi, Medium, Lo" if needed. Creating these categories involves clinical judgment so behavioral examples must be given to guide others in using these ideas.

For bulimic movement patterns used in the example, the same sort of quantification must be done. The movement patterns identified by Stark, Aronow, and McGeehan (1989) as characteristic of people with bulimia are peripheral movement, purge posture, inactive trunk, restricted use of space, exaggerated quickness and time urgency or no sense of time, loss of integrated body connections, active passive mode, and superficial affect. The researcher needs to define if these will be noted only as present or absent, as frequencies, et cetera.

If it is desired to develop a richer and more sophisticated measure of movement patterns associated with bulimia, one can make use of available validated measures. One of these is the Kestenberg Movement Profile (Kestenberg, 1965a, 1965b, 1966). This measure works within the same theoretical tradition that Chace used (Loman & Brandt, 1992). It is a comprehensive system and takes some time to learn. Once this is accomplished it is easy to calculate rating scores because Nava Lotan has created a computerized scoring program which is available at no cost on the internet (Lotan & Tziperman, 2003).

Using established sources for operational definitions has the advantage of having documentation on their reliability and validity and the high probability that there is relevant literature using the concept. If a complex concept is used, it is best to use an established system. Advanced systems take time to learn. It is not advised that one try to learn an advanced system if there is a limited amount of time to complete a study (Koch, 1998). It is even less advisable to try to create a scale and use it in the same study (see Chapter 4 in this text). Scale development takes time, has a methodological focus, and requires statistical procedures. Instrument development can stand alone as a publishable research project.

In the long run validity is necessary. In the short run reliability is what makes research proceed. The key to reliability is clearly defining basic terms. With the theory, diagnosis, and identification of dance therapy and bulimic behaviors one can now undertake a descriptive case study.

To record the data for the study a data collection instrument and a codebook are developed. The codebook is a written set of instructions, with examples, of how to record the data. Where the categories are determined by observation there needs to be a procedure, usually with the use of a second observer, to help train the primary observer so that they can reliably make behavioral judgments.

Anyone who has filled out a questionnaire where they check the alternatives understands what a data collection instrument and a codebook are. Data collected with such instruments are called pre-coded questionnaires. Such instruments often don't require written codebooks since all the necessary decisions are contained in the data collection instrument. Observational studies almost always require a written codebook since the observer needs instructions and examples to make accurate decisions.

Design

All research has variations in design and technique that are aimed at the strengths and weaknesses of a given method. There are no perfect designs or techniques. All the researcher can do is select those that are best and most practical for a given project.

The design of case study research is almost a given in that with a single case one reports on what happens with the case. If the study is to report on practice, the most usual form is to take measures on the concepts of interest before the intervention and then to repeat the measures after the intervention (Jayartane, 1978). If it is desired to chart progress repeated measures can be taken. Data for later analysis can be obtained by using video or audio tape, case notes, or original and/or standardized data collection instruments or scales.

Review of the Literature

The aim of a literature review is to justify the study (Marshall, 1999). One of the great myths about research is that each project must be unique and never have been done before (Schein, 1987). Knowledge advances by building on what is known. Even the most revolutionary theories have antecedents (Einstein, 1934). If relevant literature is not readily available it is an indication that the problem is not formulated in a way that other scholars have found useful.

One of the considerations in selecting a topic is the easy availability of relevant literature. The review is finished when new items repeat established conclusions. This points to another function of the hypothesis. It helps keep the study under control because the researchers know what to include and what to leave out of the data collection instrument.

The literature is also a good source for research ideas. Researchers usually handle the weaknesses of their study by making suggestions for future research. These offer thoughts about justification, design, established measures, data collection, and methods of analysis. They also provide a base for comparison with other findings.

Techniques

There are a large number of instruments and measurement scales that are available (Aldridge, 1994; Creswell, 1994; Fonagy & Moran, 1993; Halmii, 1996; Jayartane, 1978). There is a validated scale available for almost any concept one is interested in (Antonovsky, 1987; Buchanan, 1984; Davis, 1983; North, 1972; Northway, 1967; Sandel & Johnson, 1996). Miller's *Handbook of Research Design and Social Measurement* is an excellent source of scales and references to other books of social and psychological scales (Miller, 1991). The various types of *Mental Measurement Yearbooks* published by the Buros Institute of Mental Measurements also offer a fruitful source of instruments. Many of these sources are also available on the World Wide Web. The best way to learn a technique is to use it. Among the procedures associated with case study are observation, comparative analysis, and life history. We also briefly describe how computers can serve case study research efforts.

Observation

Observation must be systematic and recorded. It is the ultimate tool in science. Every study uses observation at some point. Observation and experiment are part of the same process since an experiment can't be done without observing the data (Kaplan, 1964). Controlled clinical experiments are not possible without case studies. It is only through case studies done before the experiment that it is possible to identify and account for possible problems and variables that might confound experimental results (Campbell, 1988; Campbell & Stanley, 1963). Laboratory researchers using the most sophisticated measuring instruments must read their data with the same observation processes that clinicians use. Sharing observations with confidence depends on knowing that trained observers will see the same things (Bartlett, 1970; Chaiklin, 1975). Excellent sources for observation procedures are found in both Junker (1960) and Wax (1971).

Comparative Analysis

Comparative analysis has been and continues to be a major technique in social science (Easthope, 1974; Ragin, 1987). It is a way to advance an argument without manipulating the data and is essential in analyzing data (Marshall, 1999). In some sense all knowledge depends on comparison (Campbell, 1989). If there were no night we would not know what day is. Skill in comparative analysis helps to avoid the tendency to want everything to be perfect and adds to confidence in presenting results where conclusions are based on a preponderance of evidence. A *DSM-IV* (1994) diagnosis depends on comparative analysis. Problem behaviors are compared to a standard in the manual. There is a primary diagnosis, a secondary diagnosis and some problem behaviors left over that can't be assigned to any category. Research results also take the same form.

Life History

Life histories are a key investigative technique in history and anthropology and a mainstay in clinical research (Becker, 1970). It is a way to see the world as the other sees it (Easthope, 1974). Recordings, observations, and field techniques used in these disciplines provide a good source of information about ways to conduct case study research (Luken & Luken, 1999; also see Chapter 9 in this volume). Classic life histories can be consulted to see how the data are organized in relation to the theory that guides their collection (Baruch, 1952; Freud, 1953; Shaw & McKay, 1972; Simmons, 1942; Thomas, 1967). Recent critiques of empiricism in research have brought renewed interest in these methodologies. Denzin (1989) calls this "interpretive interactionism" and says that it "signifies an attempt to join traditional symbolic interactionist thought with participant observation and ethnography"(p. 7).

The Computer

The computer is a boon to case study research because it permits easy collection, storing, and manipulation of data (Turner, 2002). A data set that would have required a mainframe computer and several weeks for analysis twenty years ago can now be accomplished in a few minutes with a desktop computer.

A range of computer based or amenable clinical instruments is available. They facilitate data collection and analysis. Since these instruments are in wide use their references point to literature which can support the idea under consideration. Miller's *Psychodynamic Treatment Research* has excellent sections on measuring process and outcome in psychotherapy (Miller, Luborsky, Barber, & Docherty, 1993). Specialized data analysis instruments, such as those for content analysis, expand the capability of the individual researcher. Writing aids such as spell checkers and bibliography programs that produce correct citations in a variety of styles facilitate the mechanics of writing.

The computer also has limits. There is a saying in the computer world that you should not use a computer unless you can just about solve the problem with paper and pencil. The computer is no substitute for thinking and verified clinical judgment. The computer is a tool; it only does what you tell it to do.

Data Collection

In a theory-based study the data to be collected reflect the operational definitions of the main concepts, significant factors from the review of the literature and relevant social characteristics. Simple, complete, and consistent data collection instruments should be used. Every item should be justified by the literature review. Each unnecessary variable increases the amount of time it will take to complete the study.

Inherent in developing a data collection instrument is a plan for managing it (Davis, 1971). Since a case study often collects information on a wide range of variables, it is easy to collect so much data that it proves impossible to organize. For example, if a researcher who wants to get "everything relevant" decides to record sessions, thirty hours of tapes can quickly accumulate. Without a plan for the content analysis of these data, the tapes may have to be viewed twenty times to see what "emerges." In addition, other observers then must use the system to establish its reliability.

In collecting data, often samples are drawn. One cannot, for example, record every movement and verbal expression in an hour's dance therapy session. A sample would need to be drawn. Any elementary statistics book can provide information on drawing appropriate samples, or see Cruz and Koch in this volume for information specific to sampling movement observations.

Permission

Research requires permission (Church, Shopes, & Blanchard, 2002). There are three kinds of permission and all must be secured. The first concerns getting access from those in charge of the setting where the research is to be conducted. Some thought needs to go into presenting a proposal so that permission is granted. This is where the preparation of a concise and clear proposal pays off.

The second relates to using procedures that follow mandated Federal guidelines for protecting "human subjects." In most cases research that makes no intervention in a person's life and is based on observation or collecting survey data is either exempt from the full review or is given an expedited review. If therapy is part of the case study this is an intervention and a full review is necessary.

The final permission is obtained from the patient. The patient must understand what the research is about and be free to decide whether or not they will participate in the research.

Pilot Study and Pretest

Often case studies are done as pilot studies to help decide if it is worth doing the larger study. Data from the pilot study can often be incorporated into the final study. A pilot study is different from a pretest. A pilot study is done during the development phase of the project to see if it is feasible. A pretest is used to see if instruments work. The aim is to see if the proposed method of collecting data fits the population at which it is aimed. It also helps the researcher make necessary changes to instruments and refinements in design. A little time invested in this early on in the process can save a lot of grief later.

Write Up

Guides for writing and presenting research are easily available (Barzun & Graff, 1970; Burack, 1988; Harris & Blake, 1976; Houp & Pearsall, 1968; Turabian, 1996). Textbooks provide directions on ways to both conduct and report research (Colby, 1960; Miller et al., 1993; Stake, 1995). They are guides, not exact prescriptions. Reports on the way research is actually done often show that initial outlines are discarded as necessary changes are made and a new outline is made when the project is written up for publication (Kaplan, 1964; Marshall, 1999). *The important thing is to get started and to keep working steadily.*

Even if everything has been perfectly prepared there is always some problem that crops up. If the preparation for the study has been properly done, these inevitable blows can be handled. The value of having a theoretical hypothesis is that it can be tested anywhere. If one setting is suddenly not available another one will do. If the interest is in a young person with bulimia the same case study can be done with an older person.

It seldom turns out that an hypothesis is completely supported or rejected. That is normal in all science. The researcher's obligation in writing up the final report is to tell what happened. The weaknesses in the study should be identified and there should be a statement as to how they are compensated for or how they limit the hypothesis. Unless a weakness is fatal, the reporting of these should be done positively as suggestions for future research.

ILLUSTRATION

We have chosen to illustrate the nature of the case study by presenting a therapy case that initially was seen only as a treatment situation (we also include in Appendix A a reference list of case study research that dance/movement therapists will find of interest). After the treatment was completed it was conceptualized as a case study. This will show that the relationship between treatment and practice is so close that research can be initiated at any point during treatment and that no distortion of therapy is necessary to do successful research. Please note that key facts have been changed to protect the identity of the client.

A woman in her middle thirties came asking for dance therapy. The precipitating factor was the suicide of a close friend. She had been in treatment previously for anorexia and bulimia. She was bulimic when she began this therapy and stated that she chose dance therapy because of her satisfaction with a time limited group experience a few years earlier.

She suffered with poor body image, low self-esteem, difficulty in relationships, depression and difficulty in expressing a range of feelings. These are typical characteristics of a bulimic (Stark et al., 1989, p. 121). She had many physical complaints that kept her from feeling well.

Her movement fit into many of the characteristics identified by Stark, Aronow, and McGeehan (1989). It was mostly peripheral with limited use of the trunk. While she used space, it was with superficial affect. The movement all reached upward as if not feeling the ground beneath her. It was clear from her body use that many parts of her self were ignored.

Observation was done using procedures developed by Laban and further elaborated by Lamb (Laban, 1960; Lamb, 1965). The dance therapist worked from a Chacian theoretical base which emphasized concepts of body action, therapeutic movement relationship and symbolism which culminate in the movement synchrony which is so important in establishing a trusting relationship.

She describes the treatment as follows:

I moved with the client, following the patterns of movement easily available to her, attuning to her timing, space and use of weight. At times new movement was introduced for brief moments in order to offer alternate possibilities and a reciprocal relationship became possible. By enabling the client to feel comfortable in being seen in what was available to her, the fear of judgment diminished. This led to her being able to move on her own. However, there were many weeks of movement that took on aspects of being a "good little girl" as she twirled and did sweeping movement that seemed distant from her inner self and feelings.

As more focus was given to the body, there were many sessions of limited movement. She struggled to find how to move her shoulders, her hips, her feet. It was when she finally allowed herself to get into a sense of her own body that she began to make some significant changes. With great difficulty, she experienced rage and anger. It is still something that remains hard for her to do. Her self-esteem has gradually improved as she has developed more a sense of self. Her movement changed from the upward twirling and held torso to more groundedness and sequential movement using different segments of the body. She is no longer bulimic.

Discussion

The therapist, an experienced clinician, was well versed in the Chace technique and a competent observer of behavior patterns (Samuels, 1972). She worked from a Chacian theoretical base which emphasized concepts of body action, therapeutic movement relationship, and symbolism which culminate in the movement synchrony which is so important in establishing a trusting relationship. While the therapy was undertaken with the expectation of a positive outcome, no guarantees were given to the client, nor should they have been. Even though it was unintended, the therapy had the structure of an exploratory study since the aim was to see if there would be a relationship between the Chace method of therapy and change in her movement patterns. The course of this therapy is summarized in Table 5-I by using the categories identified by Stark, Aronow, and McGeehan (1989). In most areas, except purge posture which was low to begin with, there was some improvement. The conclusion was that there was support for the hypothesis.

The therapist was not accustomed to thinking in terms of numerical ratings but with a little thought was able to make judgments. Since the number ratings in Table 5-I do not reflect judgments against a normed scale they should be considered relative. The table reflects a good way to present a summary view of what happened between the beginning and the end of therapy.

Table 5-I   CHANGE IN MOVEMENT CHARACTERISTICS
OVER THE COURSE OF THERAPY

Movement Characteristics	Beginning	End
Peripheral movement	8	4
Purge posture	2	2
Inactive trunk	8	3
Restricted use of space	5	3
Exaggerated quickness and time urgency	7	5
Loss of integrated body connections	7	3
Active passive mode	5	4
Superficial affect	9	7

Note: Higher numbers indicate a negative characteristic.

It should be noted that while a high score is a negative feature, the goal was not to seek perfection. All people display these patterns to some extent. Work could be done to norm these scores so that one would have an idea of when a behavior pattern was so discrepant that it indicated that there was some disturbance in the person.

While the therapy was not undertaken as a case study it could be written up and presented as one. If enough case studies like this were done it might be possible to develop some understanding of what the best treatment approach for bulimia is and what is an optimal behavior pattern in the dimensions examined.

CONCLUSION

In this paper we have said that the ability to do a case study is something that does not require advanced or complex statistics and methods. Rather, it requires that one be bothered enough by something to want to find out about it. Once one has that "divine itch," observing, operationalizing and presenting data flow naturally. Further, we have stressed that it helps to make the study theory based. Polansky sums this up by saying that theory is practical, saves energy, focuses energy, and makes us persuasive and able to act with certainty (Polansky, 1986). Case study research can make a contribution to helping people, professional learning, and furthering dance therapy as a profession. It has been said that "The greatest way to learn is to teach." Research is self-teaching.

Authors' Note. Thanks are due to Sharon Goodill, Sandra Holloway, and Kathryn Clough for their careful reading and judicious comments.

REFERENCES

Aldridge, D. (1994). Single-case research designs for the creative arts therapist. *The Arts in Psychotherapy, 21*(5), 333–342.

American Psychiatric Association. (1994). *Diagnostic and statistical manual of mental disorders* (4th ed.). Washington, DC: Author.

Antonovsky, A. (1987). *Unraveling the mystery of health: How people manage stress and stay well.* San Francisco, CA: Jossey-Bass.

Argyris, C., & Schön, D. A. (1974). *Theory in practice: Increasing professional effectiveness.* San Francisco, CA: Jossey-Bass.

Axline, V. M. (1964). *Dibs in search of self.* New York: Ballantine Books.

Bartlett, H. M. (1970). *The common base of social work.* Washington, DC: National Association of Social Workers.

Baruch, D. W. (1952). *One little boy.* New York: Dell.

Barzun, J., & Graff, H. F. (1970). *The modern researcher* (Revised ed.). New York: Harcourt, Brace & World.

Becker, H. S. (1958). Problems of inference and proof in participant observation. *American Sociological Review, 23*(6), 652–660.

Becker, H. S. (1970). The relevance of life histories. In N. K. Denzin (Ed.), *Sociological methods: A sourcebook.* Chicago, IL: Aldine Publishing.

Bernard, C. (1949). *An introduction to the study of experimental medicine.* New York: Henry Schuman.

Berrol, C. F. (2000). The spectrum of research options in dance/movement therapy. *American Journal of Dance Therapy, 22*(1), 29–46.

Bruch, H. (1974). *Learning psychotherapy.* Cambridge, MA: Harvard University Press.

Buchanan, D. R. (1984). Moreno's social atom: A diagnostic and treatment tool for exploring interpersonal relationships. *The Arts in Psychotherapy, 11*(3), 155–164.

Burack, S. K. (Ed.). (1988). *The writer's handbook.* Boston, MA: The Writer.

Campbell, D. T. (1988). *Methodology and epistemology for social science: Collected papers.* E. S. Overman (Ed.). Chicago, IL: University of Chicago Press.

Campbell, D. T. (1989). *Foreword to case study research, by Robert K. Yin.* Newbury Park, CA: Sage.

Campbell, D. T., & Stanley, J. C. (1963). *Experimental and quasi-experimental designs for research.* Chicago, IL: Rand McNally College Publishing.

Chaiklin, H. (1968). *Research and the development of a profession.* Paper presented at the Third Annual Meeting of the American Dance Therapy Association, Madison, Wisconsin.

Chaiklin, H. (1975). *Multiple theoretical perspectives in interpreting behavior.* Paper presented at the Ninth Annual Conference American Dance Therapy Association.

Chaiklin, H. (1997). Research and the development of a profession revisited. *American Journal of Dance Therapy, 19*(2), 93–103.

Chaiklin, S., & Schmais, C. (1993). The Chace approach to dance therapy. In S. L. Sandel, S. Chaiklin, & A. Lohn (Eds.), *Foundations of dance/movement therapy: The life and work of Marian Chace* (pp. 75–97). Columbia, MD: The Marian Chace Memorial Fund.

Charlton, B. G., & Walston, F. (1998). Individual case studies in clinical research. *Journal of Evaluation in Clinical Practice, 4*(2), 147–155.

Church, J. T., Shopes, L., & Blanchard, M. (2002). Should all disciplines be subject to the common rule? Human subjects of social science research. *Academe, 88,* 62–69.

Cohen, M. R., & Nagel, E. (1934). *An introduction to logic and scientific method.* New York: Harcourt, Brace & Company.

Colby, K. M. (1960). *An introduction to psychoanalytic research.* New York: Basic Books.

Creswell, J.W. (1994). *Research design: Qualitative & quantitative approaches.* Thousand Oaks, CA: Sage.

Cruz, R. F., & Sabers, D. L. (1998). Letter: Dance/movement therapy is more effective than previously reported. *The Arts in Psychotherapy, 25*(2), 101–103.

Davis, J. A. (1971). *Elementary survey analysis.* Englewood Cliffs, NJ: Prentice-Hall.

Davis, M. (1983). An introduction to the Davis nonverbal communication analysis system (DaNCAS). *American Journal of Dance Therapy, 6,* 49–73.

Denzin, N. K. (1989). *Interpretive interactionism.* Newbury Park, CA: Sage.

Derogatis, L. R. (1977). *SCL-90 : administration, scoring & procedures manual for the R (Revised) version and other instruments of the psychopathology rating scale series.* Baltimore: Johns Hopkins Medical School.

Easthope, G. (1974). *History of social research methods.* London: Longman.

Eckstein, H. (2000). Case study and theory in political science. In R. Gomm & M. Hammersley & P. Foster (Eds.), *Case study method* (pp. 119-164). London: Sage.

Edwards, J. (1999). Considering the paradigmatic frame: Social science research approaches relevant to research in music therapy. *The Arts in Psychotherapy, 26*(2), 73–80.

Einstein, A. (1934). *Essays in science.* New York: Philosophical Library.

Erikson, E. H. (1959). The nature of clinical evidence. In D. Lerner (Ed.), *Evidence and inference.* Glencoe, IL: The Free Press.

Erikson, E. H. (1968). *Identity youth and crisis.* New York: W.W. Norton & Company.

Erikson, E. H. (1975). *Life history and the historical moment.* New York: W.W. Norton & Company.

Feigl, H. (1945). Operationism and scientific method. *The Psychological Review, 52*(5), 250–258.

Fisch, M. H. (1986). *Peirce, semiotic, and pragmatism.* Bloomington, IN: Indiana University Press.

Fisher, S., & Greenberg, R. P. (Eds.). (1997). *From placebo to panacea: Putting psychiatric drugs to the test.* New York: John Wiley & Sons.

Fonagy, P., & Moran, G. (1993). Selecting single case research designs for clinicians. In N. E. Miller, L. Luborsky, J. P. Barber, & J. P. Docherty (Eds.), *Psychodynamic treatment research: A handbook for clinical practice* (pp. 62–95). New York: Basic Books.

Freud, A. (1971). Foreword. In M. Gardiner (Ed.), *The wolf-man: By the wolf-man.* New York: Basic Books.

Freud, S. (1953). *Collected papers* (Vol. III). London: The Hogarth Press.

Galliher, J. F. (2002). What they said and what they did: Some early SSSP presidents. *Social Problems, 49*(1), 1–10.

Gilgun, J. F. (1994). A case for case studies in social work research. *Social Work, 39*(4), 371–380.

Gomm, R., Hammersley, M., & Foster, P. (Eds.). (2000). *Case study methods.* Thousand Oaks, CA: Sage.

Good, C. V., & Scates, D. E. (1954). *Methods of research.* New York: Appleton-Century Crofts.

Gottman, J. M., & Leiblum, S. R. (1974). *How to do psychotherapy and how to evaluate it.* New York: Holt, Rinehart and Winston.

Hall, S. S. (2002, December 1). Mapping the heavens, curing dandruff. *The New York Times,* pp. 13–14.

Halmii, A. (1996). The qualitative approach to social work: An epistemological basis. *International Social Work, 39,* 363–375.

Hammersley, M., & Gomm, R. (2000). Introduction. In R. Gomm, M. Hammersley, & P. Foster (Eds.), *Case study method* (pp. 1–16). London: Sage.

Harris, J. S., & Blake, R. H. (1976). *Technical writing for social scientists.* Chicago, IL: Nelson Hall.

Herreid, C. F., & Schiller, N. A. (1999). *Case studies.* Retrieved June 15, 1999, from the World Wide Web: http://ublib.buffalo.edu/libraries/projects/cases/case.html.

Higgens, L. (2001). On the value of conducting dance/movement therapy research. *The Arts in Psychotherapy, 28*(3), 191–195.

Holt, R. R. (1961). Clinical judgment as a disciplined inquiry. *The Journal of Nervous and Mental Disease, 133*(5), 369–382.

Houp, K. W., & Pearsall, T. E. (1968). *Reporting technical information.* Beverly Hills, CA: Glencoe Press.

Innes, M. A., Greenfield, S. M., & Greenfield, M. H. (2000). Using case studies for prescribing research—an example from homeopathic prescribing. *Journal of Clinical Pharmacy and Therapeutics, 25,* 399–409.

Jahoda, M., Deutsch, M., & Cook, S. W. (1951). *Research methods in social relations: Basic processes.* (Vol. 1). New York: Dryden Press.

Jayartane, S. (1978). Analytic procedures for single-subject designs. *Social Work Research and Abstracts, 14,* 30–40.

Johnson, Y. M. (1997). Scientist-practitioner: Remaining holes in the debate. *Social Work Research, 21*(3), 196–199.

Junker, B. H. (1960). *Field work: An introduction to the social sciences.* Chicago, IL: University of Chicago Press.

Kaplan, A. (1964). *The conduct of inquiry: Methodology for behavioral science.* San Francisco, CA: Chandler Publishing.

Kassier, J. P. (1983). Teaching clinical medicine by iterative hypothesis testing. *The New England Journal of Medicine, 309*(15), 921–923.

Kestenberg, J. S. (1965a). The role of movement patterns in development: 1. rhythms of movement. *Psychoanalytic Quarterly, 34,* 1–36.

Kestenberg, J. S. (1965b). The role of movement patterns in development: 2. flow of tension and effort. *Psychoanalytic Quarterly, 34,* 517-563.

Kestenberg, J. S. (1966). The role of movement patterns in development: 3. the control of shape. *Psychoanalytic Quarterly, 36,* 356–409.

Koch, S. (1998). The Kestenberg movement profile analysis program. *American Journal of Dance Therapy, 20*(1), 57–60.

Laban, R. (1960). *Mastery of movement.* London: MacDonald & Evans.

Lamb, W. (1965). *Posture and gesture.* London: Gerald Duckworth.

Loman, S., & Brandt, R. (1992). *The body mind connection in human movement analysis.* Keene, NH: Antioch New England Graduate School.

Lotan, N., & Tziperman, E. (2003). *The Kestenberg movement profile analysis program.* Retrieved January 7, 2003, from the World Wide Web: www.weizmann.ac.il/ESER/People/Eli/KMP/home.html.

Luken, P. C., & Luken, P. C. (1999). Life history and the critique of American sociological practice. *Sociological Inquiry, 69*(3), 404–425.

Lynd, R. S., & Lynd, H. M. (1929). *Middletown: A study in American culture.* New York: Harcourt, Brace & Company.

Manpower and training for corrections. (1964, 1966). Paper presented at the Arden House Conference on Manpower and Training for Corrections, New York.

Marshall, V. W. (1999). Reasoning with case studies: Issues in an aging workforce. *Journal of Aging Studies, 13*(4), 377–389.

McCall, G. J., & Simmons, J. (Eds.). (1969). *Issues in participant observation.* Boston, MA: Addison-Wesley.

Meehl, P. E. (1954). *Clinical vs. statistical prediction.* Minneapolis, MN: University of Minnesota Press.

Merton, R. K. (1957). The self-fulfilling prophecy. In R. K. Merton (Ed.), *Social theory and social structure* (Revised ed., pp. 421–436). Glencoe, IL: The Free Press.

Mill, J. S. (1988). *The logic of the moral sciences.* La Salle, IL: Open Court.

Miller, D. C. (Ed.). (1991). *Handbook of research design and social measurement* (5th ed.). Newbury Park, CA: Sage.

Miller, N. E., Luborsky, L., Barber, J. P., & Docherty, J. P. (Eds.). (1993). *Psychodynamic treatment research: A handbook for clinical practice.* New York: Basic Books.

Mitchell, J. C. (2000). Case and situation analysis. In R. Gomm & M. Hammersley & P. Foster (Eds.), *Case study method* (pp. 165–186). London: Sage.

Nagel, E. (1961). *The structure of science.* New York: Harcourt, Brace & World.

North, M. (1972). *Personality assessment through movement.* London: Macdonald & Evans Ltd.

Northway, M. L. (1967). *A primer of sociometry* (2nd ed.). Toronto: University of Toronto Press.

Polansky, N. A. (1986). There is nothing so practical as a good theory. *Child Welfare, LXV,* 3–15.

Popper, K. R. (1965). *The logic of scientific discovery.* New York: Harper Torchbooks.

Proctor, E. K. (2001). Building and consolidating knowledge for practice. *Social Work Research, 25*(4), 195–197.

Ragin, C. C. (1987). *The comparative method: Moving beyond qualitative and quantitative strategies.* Berkeley, CA: University of California Press.

Ragin, C. C., & Becker, H. S. (Eds.). (1992). *What is a case? Exploring the foundations of social inquiry.* New York: Cambridge University Press.

Reynolds, P. D. (1971). *A primer in theory construction.* Indianapolis, IN: The Bobbs-Merrill Company.

Riley, M. W., & Nelson, E. E. (Eds.). (1974). *Sociological observation: A strategy for new knowledge.* New York: Basic Books.

Ritter, M., & Low, K. G. (1996). Effects of dance movement therapy: A meta-analysis. *The Arts in Psychotherapy, 23*(3), 249–259.

Ruddock, R. (Ed.). (1972). *Six approaches to the person.* Boston, MA: Routledge & Kegan Paul.

Samuels, A. S. (1972). Movement change through dance therapy—a study. *Writings on body movement and communication: Monograph 2* (pp. 50–72). Columbia, MD: American Dance Therapy Association.

Sandel, S. L., Chaiklin, S., & Lohn, A. (Eds.). (1993). *Foundations of dance movement therapy: The life and work of Marian Chace.* Columbia, MD: The Marian Chace Memorial Fund.

Sandel, S. L., & Johnson, D. R. (1996). Theoretical foundations of the structural analysis of movement sessions. *The Arts in Psychotherapy, 23*(1), 15–25.

Schein, E. H. (1987). *The clinical perspective in fieldwork* (Vol. 5). Newbury Park, CA: Sage.

Schön, D. A. (1983). *The reflective practitioner: How professionals think in action.* New York: Basic Books.

Shapiro, A. K., & Shapiro, A. K. (1997). *The powerful placebo: From ancient priest to modern physician.* Baltimore, MD: The Johns Hopkins University Press.

Shaw, C. R., & McKay, H. D. (1972). *Juvenile delinquency and urban areas* (Revised ed.). Chicago, IL: The University of Chicago Press.

Siegel, E. V. (1993). Marian Chace and psychoanalysis. In S. L. Sandel, S. Chaiklin, & A. Lohn (Eds.), *Foundations of dance/movement therapy: The life and work of Marian Chace* (pp. 169–175). Columbia, MD: The Marian Chace Memorial Fund.

Simmons, L. W. (1942). *Sun chief: The autobiography of a Hopi Indian.* New Haven, CT: Yale University Press.

Skagestad, P. (1981). *The road of inquiry: Charles Peirce's pragmatic realism.* New York: Columbia University Press.

Smitskamp, H. (1995). The problem of professional diagnosis in the arts therapies. *The Arts in Psychotherapy, 22*(3), 181–187.

Spence, D. P. (1993). Traditional case studies and prescriptions for improving them. In N. E. Miller, L. Luborsky, J. P. Barber, & J. P. Docherty (Eds.), *Psychodynamic treatment research: A handbook for clinical practice* (pp. 37–52). New York: Basic Books.

Stake, R. E. (1995). *The art of case study research.* Thousand Oaks, CA: Sage.

Stark, A., Aronow, S., & McGeehan, T. (1989). Dance/movement therapy with bulimic patients. In L. M. Hornyak & E. K. Baker (Eds.), *Experiential therapies for eating disorders* (pp. 121–143). New York: The Guilford Press.

Stefanek, M. E., Derogartis, L. P., & Shaw, A. (1993). Psychological distress among oncology outpatients: Prevalence and severity as measured with the Brief Symptom Inventory. *Psychosomatics, 28,* 530–532.

Thomas, W. I. (1967). *The unadjusted girl.* New York: Harper Torchbooks.

Tuckett, A. (1999). Bending the truth: professional narratives about lying and deception in nursing practice. *International Journal of Nursing Studies, 35*(5), 292–302.

Turabian, K. L. (1996). *A manual for writers of term papers, theses, and dissertations* (6th ed., Revised by John Grossman and Alice Bennett Eds.). Chicago, IL: The University of Chicago Press.

Turner, F. J. (2002). *Diagnosis in social work: New imperatives.* New York: The Haworth Social Work Practice Press.

Wax, R. (1971). *Doing fieldwork: Warnings and advice.* Chicago, IL: University of Chicago Press.

Yin, R. K. (1989). *Case study research: Design and methods* (Revised ed.). Newbury Park, CA: Sage.

Zabora, J., Szoc, K., Jacobsen, P., Curbow, B., Piantadosi, S., Hooker, C., et al. (2001). A new psychosocial screening instrument for use with cancer patients. *Psychosomatics, 42*(3), 241–248.

Appendix A

EXAMPLES OF THE CASE STUDY
IN CURRENT LITERATURE

Ben-Asher, S., & Koren, B. (2002). Case study of a five year-old Israeli girl in movement therapy. *American Journal of Dance Therapy, 24*(1), 27–33.

Blumberg, S., & Coche, E. (1980). The use of movement in a psychotherapy group. *American Journal of Dance Therapy, 3*(2), 56–64.

Burton, C. L., & Ancelin-Schutzenberger, A. (1977). Nonverbal communication in the verbal and nonverbal interaction: A research approach. *American Journal of Dance Therapy, 1*(1), 20–24.

Cohen, B. M. (1983). Combined art and movement therapy group: Isomorphic responses. *The Arts in Psychotherapy, 10*(4), 229–232.

Cole, I. L. (1982). Movement negotiations with an autistic child. *The Arts in Psychotherapy, 9*(1), 49–53.

Davis, M., Walters, S. B., Vorus, N., & Connors, B. (2000). Defensive demeanor profiles. *American Journal of Dance Therapy, 22*(2), 103–121.

Dendinger, R. A., & Trop, J. L. (1979). Combined physical and psychiatric disability: A case study in movement therapy. *American Journal of Dance Therapy, 3*(1), 15–19.

Fiasca, P. M. (1993). A research study on anxiety and movement. *American Journal of Dance Therapy, 15*(2), 89–105.

Fraenkel, D. L. (2002). Moving dance/movement therapy from isolation to integration. *American Journal of Dance Therapy, 24*(1), 37–43.

Frank, Z. (1997). Dance and expressive movement therapy: An effective treatment for a sexually abused man. *American Journal of Dance Therapy, 19*(1), 45–61.

Frost, M. C. S. (1984). Changing movement patterns and lifestyle in a blind obsessive compulsive. *American Journal of Dance Therapy, 7*, 15–31.

Ginzberg, J. (1991). In search of a voice: Working with homeless men. *American Journal of Dance Therapy, 13*(1), 33–48.

Goodill, S. W. (1983). Dance/movement therapy with abused children. *The Arts in Psychotherapy, 14*(1), 59–68.

Gordon-Cohen, N. (1987). Vietnam and reality—the story of Mr. D. *American Journal of Dance Therapy, 10*, 95–109.

Gray, A. E. (2001). The body remembers: Dance/movement therapy with an adult survivor of torture. *American Journal of Dance Therapy, 23*(1), 29–43.

Lett, W. R. (1998). Researching experiential self-knowing. *The Arts in Psychotherapy, 25*(5), 331–342.

Lewin, J. L. N. (1999). *Dance therapy notebook.* Columbia, MD: The Marian Chace Foundation.

Loughlin, E. E. (1993). "Why was I born among mirrors?" Therapeutic dance for teenage girls and women with Turner Syndrome. *American Journal of Dance Therapy, 15*(2), 107–124.

McIntosh, J., E. (2002). Thought in the face of violence: A child's need. *Child Abuse and Neglect, 26*, 229–241.

Mendelsohn, J. (1999). Dance/movement therapy with hospitalized children. *American Journal of Dance Therapy, 21*(2), 65–80.

Ostrov, K. S. (1981). A movement approach to the study of infant/caregiver communication during infant psychotherapy. *American Journal of Dance Therapy, 4*(1), 25–41.

Perowsky, G. (1991). Working with pain: A self-study. *American Journal of Dance Therapy, 13*(1), 49–58.

Rossberg-Gempton, I., & Poole, G. D. (1992). The relationship between body movement and affect from historical and current perspectives. *The Arts in Psychotherapy, 19*(1), 39–46.

Scott, E. H. (1999). The body as testament: A phenomenological case study of an adult woman who self-mutilates. *The Arts in Psychotherapy, 26*(3), 149–164.

Sommer, R., Motley, J. C., & Cassandro, V. J. (1998). Perceived psychopathology in Richard Dadd's art. *The Arts in Psychotherapy, 25*(5), 323\–329.

Tropea, E. B. (2002). Discussion: Case study of a five-year-old in movement therapy: One clinician's perspective. *American Journal of Dance Therapy, 24*(1), 33–37.

Zagelbaum, V. N., & Rubina, M. A. (1991). Combined dance/movement, art and music therapies with a developmentally delayed, psychiatric client in a day treatment setting. *The Arts in Psychotherapy, 18*(2), 139–148.

Chapter 6

SINGLE-SUBJECT DESIGNS IN CLINICAL DANCE/MOVEMENT THERAPY RESEARCH

Sherry W. Goodill and Robyn Flaum Cruz

INTRODUCTION

In many situations, a dance/movement therapist may wish to evaluate the effects of introducing an intervention into the treatment of a particular individual. For example, the therapist might want to examine if introducing dance/movement therapy (DMT) into the treatment of a child with an expressive language disorder produces a corresponding increase in the child's verbal fluency. Demonstrating such a relationship might allow the therapist to argue for the inclusion of dance/movement therapy in the child's individual treatment plan, serve as an important indicator of treatment response when reporting on the child's progress to the treatment team, or if published, provide needed research information to other dance/movement therapists.

As we present and discuss in this chapter, single-subject design (SSD) studies offer an experimental research option that allows treatment issues to be investigated and provides specific answers to questions about treatment effectiveness. Studies using SSD have truly pragmatic potential for dance/movement therapy research, and we offer examples in this chapter to illustrate this point. Few dance/movement therapists have used the SSD to date. This may be due to the association of the SSD with applied behavior analysis, an area influenced by behavior modification and the work of B. F. Skinner (Baer, Wolfe, & Risley, 1968; Kazdin, 1982), which might be viewed as "at odds" with the psychodynamic approach incorporated into dance/movement therapy early in its development and used by many practitioners today.

Nevertheless, the SSD has great potential for research in dance/movement therapy, and this chapter addresses the usefulness of this method by describing the major features and benefits of SSD studies and providing a comparison with case study research. Basic procedures for carrying out SSD projects in dance/movement therapy are given, and three example studies are presented.

WHAT IS SINGLE-SUBJECT DESIGN RESEARCH?

Single-subject design studies are known by several names: single-partici-pant designs, single case designs, single case experimental designs, N = 1 studies, and intrasubject designs (Kazdin, 1982, 1992; Morgan & Morgan, 2001). In this chapter, we have chosen to use the term single-subject design, or SSD. However, the word "participant" will sometimes be substituted for the word "subject," in keeping with current conventions in the human and behavioral sciences. The SSD study is empirical in nature, meaning that data are "based on observation or experience" and findings "can be verified by observation or experience" (Vogt, 1999, p. 95).

Single-subject designs do seek to demonstrate treatment effectiveness and establish causation to some degree (Jones, 1993; Kiene & von Schön-Angerer, 1998). The main features of these designs are: a) comparison across condi-tions; b) continuous assessment; and c) data analysis through visual inspec-tion. Comparison of alternating conditions is the key to efficacy research. In group studies of therapy effectiveness, one group is given the treatment under question and compared to another, or to several other control groups that receive either no treatment, standard care, or a different treatment. This is the typical and familiar "randomized controlled clinical trial" method on which much of modern health care science has been based. In SSD research, the subject is compared to him- or herself in the different experimental con-ditions or phases of the study. Thus, *the subject serves as his or her own control,* in contrast to the standard, that is, a comparison to other individuals.

SSD studies are considered experimental or quasi-experimental, depend-ing on the specific design elements and how much control the researcher exerts over events and variables in the case (Kazdin, 1992). This approach has the potential for high internal validity, meaning that it creates positive conditions for ruling out competing hypotheses for the observed treatment effect and indeed, SSD researchers strive for internal validity. As with all forms of case study, the SSD has poor external validity, meaning that find-ings from an SSD study cannot be generalized to the population from which the study participant(s) come.

Comparison with Clinical Case Study

SSD studies are often presented as variations on the case study, and the single-subject design is indeed a form of case study. Both define a single case, or "one unit," as the focus of inquiry, and both appreciate the fact that "one" does not necessarily refer to one individual person. The term can mean a family (when studied as a system or unit), a group, a society, or a work team (Stake, 1994).

In practice, SSD projects are often conducted with more than one indi-vidual unit or case. The study protocols are carefully planned and replicable, and in fact, replication of the SSD study with several cases is encouraged. Authorities on single-subject research agree that replication of SSD studies and accumulation of cases is preferred over attempts to aggregate data from SSD studies into group-like forms (Barlow & Hersen, 1984; Hilliard, 1993).

Both SSD and traditional case study research embrace the premise that change occurs over time, and so information is collected and findings are reported with an emphasis on change as it evolves in the course of therapy and the life of the patient or subject. For the clinical researcher who wishes to investigate at the level of the single case, a look at how SSDs differ from clinical case studies (see Chapter 5, Chaiklin & Chaiklin, in this text) will inform the choice of study approaches.

Unlike the author of a case study, who may decide to investigate the case for research purposes at the beginning, middle, or end of the treatment process, the SSD researcher conceives of and enters the treatment process with research in mind. Dependent or target variables (i.e., the behaviors or characteristics the therapy aims to influence) are identified, measured and collected from the beginning of the study, including the phase before treatment begins. The case study researcher is likely to study a course of therapy as it would unfold even if it were not under investigation. In contrast, the SSD researcher deliberately manipulates certain aspects of the participant's experience (in the intervention, the data collection, or both). Because of this, most SSD studies will need to be approved by an institutional human subjects review committee. While the clinical case study may be qualitative in nature and use narrative and/or artistic data exclusively, the single-subject design study will almost always include quantitative data.

General Features of Single-Subject Designs Basic Structure

The ABA format is the prototype for SSD studies (Barlow & Hersen, 1984). The first "A" refers to the initial baseline phase: a period of observation and data collection that precedes the treatment. "B" refers to the intervention phase of the study when the treatment is introduced, and the second "A" stands for the second baseline or phase of observation. The second "A" phase is also referred to as the reversal phase, as the researcher expects the behavior observed to revert to levels similar to those of the first baseline phase. Comparison across conditions is possible only when clear and different study phases or conditions are built into the design.

The baseline phase may consist of no treatment at all, or standard care. When a new therapy is introduced into an ongoing program of several treatment components, standard care or the basic program can constitute the baseline condition. This is a common situation for many dance/movement therapists working on multidisciplinary treatment teams. When dance/movement therapy is already part of the standard care package, the study could vary the way DMT is usually provided such that the intervention being studied is sufficiently different from standard care and a comparison is feasible and relevant. For example, if a child with an expressive language disorder receives a treatment package that includes speech therapy and occupational therapy twice per week, and dance/movement therapy once per week, increasing dance/movement therapy to five times per week while the other treatments remain at the same frequency creates a condition quite different from standard care. This new therapy regimen could be used as the treatment condition. Examples of other aspects of care that could be varied are length of sessions, the inclusion of particular props, or specific movement interventions.

The purpose of the baseline phase is twofold: 1) to describe the existing level of functioning in relation to the target behavior or characteristic of interest; and 2) to establish a pattern of behavior that can predict how that behavior might naturally continue should there be no intervention (Kazdin, 1982). Thus, the first baseline phase must be long enough, and contain observations continuous enough to enable such a prediction. Important features of baseline data are the stability of the data and the trends observed in that phase. When quantitative data are plotted on a line graph, trends appear as clear slopes in the lines. The baseline pattern could be stable (indicating little or no change in the variable); or it could show a deterioration of functioning (a trend that treatment would aim to reverse), an improvement in functioning (in which case treatment would aim to increase the rate of improvement), or erratic fluctuations (which makes predictions more difficult to generate).

During the intervention, or "B" phase, observations of the target behavior or characteristic continue with the same frequency as during the first baseline phase. In addition, it is best that careful documentation of the intervention is made during this phase. The many options for types of data and ways of collecting them are discussed below.

In the second baseline phase, the final "A" of the ABA pattern, the intervention is withdrawn, and data collection continues with study conditions resembling those of the first "A" phase. This phase may be of the same duration as the initial baseline phase, shorter, or longer, depending on the target variable and the researcher's goals for the study.

Many variations on the ABA format exist. In these variations, "A" always stands for the baseline phase and "B" for the intervention phase. Here we describe a few of the more commonly seen variations. These include AB, ABAB, multiple baseline and alternating treatment designs. When multiple treatment phases or alternating treatments are used, the "A" "B" notation is extended to accommodate the design. While there are no standard conventions, frequently, alternating baselines will be noted as A1 A2 , et cetera, and alternating phases of the same treatment intervention will use similar notation while alternate treatments (different treatments) will use additional letters of the alphabet such as "C" for the second unique treatment in a study design. In AB designs, there is only one baseline and the comparison is made between this baseline phase or measurement and measurements taken during the treatment phase—a situation that is not as strong for arguing internal validity of the study or that the treatment is responsible for observed changes in target behaviors.

Sometimes the cessation of a beneficial treatment can have troublesome ethical implications. To address this, the ABA format is modified to an ABAB model: baseline–intervention–baseline–intervention. In this model, the study ends with an intervention phase, and if further treatment is indicated, it can continue without dismantling the research study.

In an alternating treatment design, the two or more interventions are alternated or scheduled sequentially through time, and both might be compared to no-treatment baseline phases. This kind of single subject research asks and answers questions such as, "Is DMT more effective than Therapy X for influencing Target Variable Y?"

Multiple baseline single subject designs involve more than one intervention and/or more than one subject in the same study (Kazdin, 1982). Note that while multiple baseline designs are useful for comparing interventions and involving more than one subject in a study, they are not equivalent to replicating a study with one subject. In a hypothetical example of a multiple baseline SSD, we (Goodill and Cruz) might devise a special short-term DMT program to increase impulse control in children with conduct disorders and implement it using SSD in a residential treatment program with four children. We would start the baseline measurements with all four of the children enrolled in the study at the same time (Week 1) for the baseline phase, but initiate the individual treatment intervention for each child at different times (Weeks 4, 6, 8 and 10 respectively). Thus, "child one" receives the treatment from Week 4 through Week 12 (eight weeks of treatment), "child two" receives the treatment from Week 6 through Week 12 (six weeks of treatment), et cetera. We return all four children to the second baseline condition at the same time (Week 13). This strategy allows us to see if a different "dose" of DMT (length of treatment) makes a difference in the rate of change or the maintenance of progress (also see Cruz's discussion in Chapter 10 of this text). Because the children started the program at different times, we can be assured that any observed effect came from the DMT and not from some other event or process in their milieu. Procedures like these enhance the internal validity of the study.

Data Collection and Other Procedures

Continuous data collection, also called continuous assessment, is a key ingredient in SSD research (Kazdin, 1982). Observations or measurements must be made repeatedly and regularly over time, preferably daily or several times per week beginning in the baseline (A) phase, continuing at the same rate during the intervention (B) phase, and the second baseline (A) phase. It is important that the conditions or context of the observation are always the same during baseline and intervention phases. The concept of serial dependency is relevant to the SSD practice of repeated measures and continuous data collection. Serial dependency is the notion that data collected from a subject over time will be meaningful only when one considers the influence that a behavior or event will have over subsequent behaviors. As Morgan and Morgan (2001) put it,

> Repeated measures are considered a natural consequence of an epistemology that conceptualizes behavior as a continuously unfolding phenomenon. Behavior exhibits considerable serial dependence, and to be scientifically viable, observational and measurement schemes must make sufficient contact with this dimension of the subject matter (p. 122).

Triangulation of data sources is advised for qualitative case study (Stake, 1994) but the use of multiple sources of data will strengthen the experimental or quasi-experimental single-subject study as well. The clinician's field notes comprise an essential data source. As Aldridge noted, "single-case designs allow for a close analysis of the therapist-patient interaction" (1994, p. 333), and dance/movement therapy notes typically convey the stream of interaction in a session. When taken consistently and in a systematic way, clinical notes provide ample documentation and description of the intervention. The SSD tradition has been built on the study of cognitive and behavioral therapies that usually have standardized clinical protocols, often for short-term interventions. However, DMT is a flexible therapy that is responsive to the needs of the patient and unfolds over time. Rich, careful description of the intervention becomes more important when studying the efficacy of a process oriented modality such as dance/movement therapy because the intervention will not be delivered in a uniform way across subjects or across sessions. Clinical field notes are qualitative (narrative) data that can be used during data analysis to help interpret changes in the target variable(s).

SSD studies can be and often are conducted with only one source of quantified data, but they are enhanced when the researcher uses a mix of qualitative and quantitative data (also see Berrol in this text for a discussion of mixing quantitative and qualitative methods). Cook and Campbell, in their 1979 discussion of social science field experimentation and quasi-experimental research, advised, "Field experimentation should always include qualitative research to describe and illuminate the context and conditions under which research is conducted" (p. 93). Qualitative data might include material from interviews with the study participant or others in his or her life, diaries or journals kept by the participant(s), clinical records and assessments, creative expressions like poetry or descriptions of artwork or movement by the subject or by raters, or heuristic exploration of the dance/movement therapist's experience.

SSDs are strengthened enormously by the use of at least one measure for which published norms exist. This way, the subject's functioning can be evaluated in relation to the population using normative information and the study's findings can be placed alongside those of other studies in health or mental health (Kazdin, 1984). Measures selected should be sensitive to short-term change. In a group of recent DMT master's thesis studies conducted with the ABA format, several such measures have proven useful. These include: the Medical Outcomes Study Short Form-36 Health Survey (MOS SF-36 version 2; Ware & Sherbourne, 1992; used by Tatum-Fairfax, 2003), the KIDCOPE (provides a brief measure to identify coping in children and adolescents; Spirito, Stark, Grace, & Stamoulis, 1991; used by Hall, 2002), the Developmental Profile II (Alpern, Boll, & Shearer, 1989; used by Ruzic, 2002), and The Behavioral Rating Scale of Presented Self-esteem in Young Children (Haltiwanger & Harter, 1989; used by Matsuzaki, 2003).

Researcher bias can be a concern in SSD research, and even though the same person may function as both researcher and clinician for a study, there are ways to limit the influence of any bias. For the most part this means having someone else who is minimally invested in the success of the study collect the observations and data on the target variable. Systematic review of progress notes by other team members in the clinical chart is a good way to obtain continuous data from impartial observers of the subject's functioning. Colleagues can be hired or recruited to conduct interviews or fill out behavioral checklists. When videotaped material is used for movement assessment as a form of outcome data, raters should be brought in to score the parameters of interest on the videotapes. A complete discussion of rater training and data collection procedures from videotape is beyond the scope of this chapter, but these issues are discussed elsewhere in this text (see Cruz & Koch, Chapter 4). Aside from the DMT clinical field notes (which will undoubtedly contain and reflect the therapist's expectations for his or her patient's improvement) any data obtained by the DMT researcher him- or herself should be as objective as possible.

Finally, one must be careful not to overburden participants with time-consuming and demanding data collection procedures that involve self-report or guided assessment. Observational procedures can and should be made unobtrusive, so they do not interfere with the potential effects of the therapy.

Data Analysis

The primary form of data analysis in SSD studies is visual inspection of data. Data are usually displayed in line graph form, making it easy to see the pattern of change over time. The treatment is considered effective if a change is observed when, and only when, the treatment is given (Kazdin, 1992). For example, imagine a pattern that shows a stable or declining trend in desired behaviors during the first baseline (A) phase (a relatively straight horizontal line or a line sloping down to the right corner of the graph). Then, imagine a line that shows an increase in frequency of that behavior during the treatment (B) phase (a line sloping to the upper right corner of the graph). Wonderful! Perhaps the DMT worked! However, the only way the researcher can be relatively sure that the treatment brought about that desirable increase is to look at the second baseline (A) phase when the therapy is withdrawn. If the trend there shows a decrease in frequency (a slope downward approaching the level of the first baseline phase), we are more assured in inferring that the therapy "caused" the change. Readers are also directed to the visual figures that accompany studies in the next section of this chapter as examples.

If lasting change is desired or warranted by the research design and behavior targeted, the researcher can include extended baseline observations after treatment to investigate this aspect. Note that the SSD does not necessarily rule out certain threats to validity that are of concern in group designs such as, the Hawthorne effect in which participants' awareness of the experiment causes them to alter their performance. However, the ability to include alternating treatments and periods of treatment with baseline phases can assist the researcher in arguing for causation and the validity of the study. It is worth noting that whenever one argues causation in research, there are actually three basic arguments that must be sufficiently put forth for the data and the research design. These are: a) covariation—as the "cause" varies, so does the "effect;" b) temporal precedence—the "cause" must precede the "effect" in time; and c) contiguity between the cause and effect—the presumed cause and effect are events that are close in time and/or space (Cook & Campbell, 1979). For a thorough treatment of causation in experimental research related to the philosophy of science, we direct the interested reader to Cook and Campbell (pp. 10–36; 1979), whose work is frequently cited by researchers as the classic reference in this area.

In most SSD projects, clinical significance rather than statistical significance is used to make judgments about the effectiveness of the therapy investigated. However, it is possible to use statistical analysis of data for a single subject. Statistical analysis supplements visual inspection of data for SSD; it does not replace it (Kazdin, 1984). Time series analyses are one way to capture the serial influence of sequenced behaviors and models for simplified time-series analysis are available (Tyron, 1982); descriptive statistics can summarize the data collected within one study phase; and significance testing can compare the numerous observations in one phase with those of others. However, not all researchers agree that statistics are useful or even appropriate when studying a single case (Michael, 1974; Hartmann, 1974).

Replication and Accumulation

As mentioned earlier, it is better to replicate an SSD study, and to work towards an accumulation of studies, than to clump data from several SSDs together and try to treat them as group data for statistical analysis or any other purpose. Replication eventually accumulates credible information about the potential generality of the findings. There are three approaches to SSD replication, each type building on a previous and more straightforward approach: direct replication, systematic replication, and clinical replication (Barlow & Hersen, 1984). When direct replication is used, the researcher simply repeats the study with the same subject or with another subject, and this can even take place concurrently so that the two subjects are studied at the same time. If a few direct replications of an SSD yield consistent results indicating a therapeutic effect, it is time to try a systematic replication. In a systematic replication of an SSD the researcher will deliberately alter some aspect of the study: the setting, the intervention technique, the therapist, or the diagnosis of the subject, and so on. Following a series of systematic replications, a single-subject researcher could conduct a clinical replication, so named because the study embraces the mixture of elements found in a real clinical program. As defined by Barlow and Hersen, clinical replication is

> the administration by the same investigator or practitioner of a treatment package containing two or more distinct treatment procedures. These procedures would be administered in a specific setting to a series of clients presenting similar combinations of multiple behaviors and emotional problems. Obviously, this type of replication process is advanced in that it should be the end result of a systematic, technique-building applied research effort, which should take years (p. 367).

Currently, there are no published series of systematic SSD replications or the more extensive clinical replications in the field of dance/movement therapy. These are ways of harnessing the power of the single-subject study that are, with careful planning, attainable and potentially quite useful for the DMT clinical researcher.

A handful of SSD studies in DMT are available to illustrate some general principles of the method. Each has different attributes, strengths, and limitations. Like the cases themselves, they are instructive in their particularity.

EXAMPLES OF SINGLE SUBJECT DESIGN STUDIES IN DANCE/MOVEMENT THERAPY

AB Design

For a study of DMT intended to increase attention to task in a 10-year old boy with attention deficit disorder, Dulicai (1996) used the AB design. The intervention was two-pronged: 1) individual DMT sessions; and 2) activities performed at home with his mother who had been taught ways of supporting the therapeutic goals. Treatment emphasized the movement elements of space and time (Dell, 1970), and was process oriented. There were two behaviors targeted as dependent variables (time attending to homework while seated at a desk, and time attending to a fine motor task—manipulating a coin through a large maze). An objective technique, the use of a stopwatch, recorded the boy's task-time in seconds. Baseline measures were taken for a period of time before therapy began. When the intervention was begun, measurements were recorded at month 3 and month 6 of treatment when the therapy and the study ended. Figure 6-1 shows the data in line graph form. While the AB design does not permit a claim that the DMT is responsible for the dramatic change in attention to task, certainly this study, which included a substantial treatment period, provided a foundation for further study of the approach for children with attention deficit disorder (Dulicai, 1996).

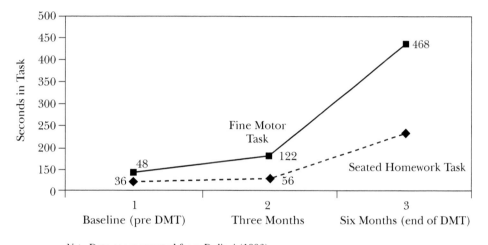

Note: Data reconstructed from Dulicai (1996).

Figure 6.1   Time (in seconds) Maintaining Attention to Task for a Boy with ADD

ABA Design

Gillern (2002) used the ABA design for an 8-week study of the effects of DMT on attachment and other relationship variables with substance abusing mothers in recovery and their preschool children. The hypothesis was that attuning behaviors such as eye contact and physical accommodation would increase with DMT treatment. The study was conducted with three mother-child dyads, using each dyad as one case. Data collection included interviews with each mother, and the clinician/researcher's clinical notes. Quantitative measurement consisted of analysis of weekly videotaped recordings of mother-child free play sessions coded with the Nonverbal Assessment of Family Systems (NVAFS, Dulicai, 1977).

The first and second baseline (A) phases lasted for two weeks, and the treatment (B) phase consisted of four weeks during which the dyads participated in twice weekly DMT sessions thirty minutes in length. Videotapes of ten-minute free play sessions were collected once per week during all study phases. A team of trained raters analyzed the videotapes using the NVAFS and noting multiple indices of attuning and separating behaviors. Reconstructed data for attuning behaviors are displayed in Figure 6-2. Only data for two of the dyads are shown as the third dyad had missing data for the second observation of the first baseline period. Symbols are used to depict the frequencies of attuning behaviors for each dyad and a linear trendline for each dyad is included in the figure simply to assist in visualization of trends (see the figure legend that defines symbols used for dyads and each dyad's trendline). The trendlines in Figure 6-2 were created with linear regression, a statistical technique used to fit a straight line through a set of observations based on the "least squares" method. A complete discussion of this technique is beyond the scope of this chapter, and we direct the statistically interested reader to Huck and Cormier (1996) or Kachigan (1991).

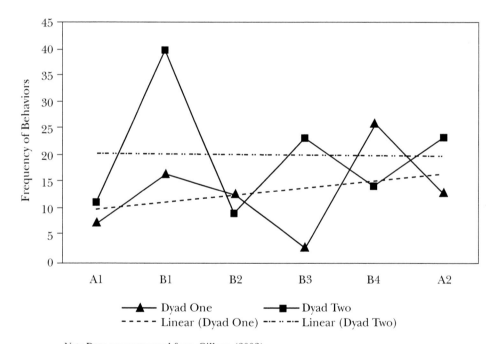

Note: Data reconstructed from Gillern (2003).

Figure 6.2 Attuning Behaviors for Two Dyads: Baseline (A) and Treatment (B) Phases

While both dyads show irregular patterns in Figure 6-2, they also show increases of attuning behaviors from the first (A1) to the second (A2) baseline. Dyad 2 shows a marked increase during the first week of treatment (B1) that was composed of high frequencies of "gesture and posture toward" and causes the regression line to have less of a marked slope than that of Dyad 1. These data are quite typical of pilot data in that they show promise but not the clear impact of treatment that is usually desired. Considering the frequency and length of treatment, and the population from which participants were selected, we interpret results to indicate that further replication is both needed and warranted for this research. A longer or more intensive treatment phase might clarify the effects of DMT with mothers in a residential substance abuse recovery program and their young children.

Multiple-baseline Design Used to Address Multiple Treatment Confound

Stewart, McMullen, and Rubin (1994) used an SSD to study effects of movement therapy with twelve depressed subjects on an inpatient psychiatric unit. A special feature of this study is that rather than using baseline and treatment phases as we have discussed thus far, each subject was randomly assigned to seven treatment (movement therapy) days and seven no-treatment (no-movement therapy) days within a fourteen-day period. Thus baseline and intervention phases (days) alternated randomly for each subject. The design was intended to control for the multiple treatment confound in that the experimental condition (movement therapy or no-movement therapy) was manipulated in the context of the full complement of therapies offered in the inpatient program. The researchers were interested in examining the immediate effects of the intervention on depressed mood. Thus, a self-report measurement of mood and depression level was taken daily from every subject at the same time: one half hour after the end of the movement therapy session regardless of group attendance.

The movement therapy intervention was a highly structured forty-five-minute group session with ten components including warm-ups, social interaction tasks, dance steps, solo and group improvisation. The sessions were not process oriented, but followed the same sequence of therapist directed activities. In this way the intervention, which derived from the nursing tradition, differed from what most dance/movement therapists might offer. Nonetheless, the study design is a good example of how SSD studies can be made experimentally rigorous. The authors noted that the randomization of movement therapy and no-movement therapy days "separated the effect of the . . . program from other coexisting interventions" (Stewart, McMullen, & Rubin, 1994, p. 28). In addition, conducting twelve replications was a prudent and creative use of resources that strengthened the external validity of the results. This study used daily measurements of the target variable (depressed mood), which meets the SSD standard of continuous assessment. The researchers statistically tested the data from each subject and found that a statistically significant reduction in depressed mood for five of the twelve participants on the movement therapy intervention days compared to the no-movement therapy days. The researchers concluded that the study "provided evidence for the antidepressant effect of MT [the treatment], as a legitimate adjunctive therapy for inpatients with unipolar depression" (p. 28).

HOW IS THE SSD USEFUL TO DANCE/MOVEMENT THERAPISTS?

There are many good reasons for dance/movement therapists to use the SSD for demonstrating the effectiveness of the therapy. Lukoff, Edwards, and Miller (1998) argued that the method is ideal for investigating complementary and alternative therapies, because they may use unique clinical practices or operate from philosophical frameworks incompatible with other research designs. Aldridge (1994) suggested that the single-subject design is ideal for asking new clinical questions. Morgan and Morgan (2001) recommend the method because the managed care system demands information on treatment effectiveness, but funds for group studies are few, and information about change is quite compelling at the individual level. Case oriented SSD is an approach that embraces the patient's uniqueness and the contexts in which he or she lives and functions. As a systematic, valid form of outcome research, it can provide convincing evidence about the benefits of DMT. Many dance/movement therapists work in programs where several therapies comprise the treatment "package." In these settings, it would be impossible and unethical to withhold other therapies in order to test the effectiveness of DMT. In classic group comparison studies, this creates a "multiple treatment confound," but single-subject experiments can successfully circumvent that challenge (Stewart, McMullen, & Rubin, 1994).

DMT is a modality that requires "systematic therapeutic learning" (Cassileth, Jonas, Cassidy et al., 1994). This means that the therapy involves a learning process, and that with experience the patient or client gradually becomes more adept with the clinical method used in treatment. In DMT, this often may mean that the client develops comfort in using movement and the body as tools of expression. Presumably then, the effectiveness of the therapy will be mediated by the amount of exposure the patient has had with DMT. These authors advised that study participants in clinical outcome research achieve a basic level of learning in the modality investigated and that studies should take into account the amount of learning among participants. When subjects are studied one at a time, we can easily record and integrate information about prior experience with the modality, and even provide a period for learning about the therapy prior to studying its effect on target variables.

This chapter serves only as an introduction to an elegant research method with a long scientific tradition. Before setting out to conduct SSD research, we recommend that the dance/movement therapist or DMT student read more extensively in one of the many authoritative texts on the topic to obtain step-by-step guidance for the wide range of procedures.

REFERENCES

Aldridge, D. (1994). Single-case research design for the creative art therapist. *Arts in Psychotherapy, 21*(5), 333–342.

Alpern, G., Boll, T., & Shearer, M. (1989). *Developmental Profile II manual.* Los Angeles, CA: Western Psychological Services.

Baer, D. M., Wolfe, M. M., & Risley, T. R. (1968). Some current dimensions of appplied behavior analysis. *Journal of Applied Behavior Analysis, 1*, 91–97.

Barlow, D. H., & Hersen, M. (1984). *Single case experimental designs: Strategies for studying behavior change.* New York: Pergamon Press.

Cassileth, B., Jonas, W., Cassidy, C. M., & others. (1994). Research methodologies. In B. M. Berman & D. B. Larson (Eds.), *Alternative medicine: Expanding medical horizons: A report to the NIH on alternative medical systems and practices in the U.S.* (pp. 289–298). Washington, DC: U.S. Government Printing Office, National Institutes of Health.

Cook, T. D., & Campbell, D. T. (1979). *Quasi-experimentation: design & analysis issues for field settings.* Chicago, IL: Rand McNally College Publishing.

Dell, C. (1970). *A primer for movement description: Using effort/shape and supplementary concepts.* New York: Dance Notation Bureau.

Dulicai, D. (1977). Nonverbal assessment of family systems: A preliminary study. *The Arts in Psychotherapy, 4*, 55–62.

Dulicai, D. (1996). *Dance/movement therapy techniques with a child with Attention Deficit Disorder.* Research poster presented at the American Dance Therapy Association/National Association of Drama Therapy Joint Conference, Santa Monica, CA.

Gillern, B. (2002). *Dance/movement therapy to repair attachment within the substance abusing mother-child dyad: A case study.* Unpublished master's thesis, Drexel University, Philadelphia, PA.

Hall, S. E. (2002). *Dance/movement therapy to improve self esteem and coping skills among African American preadolescent girls: a multiple case study.* Unpublished master's thesis, Drexel University, Philadelphia, PA.

Haltiwanger, J., & Harter, S. (Eds.). (1989). *The behavioral rating scale of presented self-esteem in young children.* Denver, CO: University of Denver.

Hartmann, D. P. (1974). Forcing square pegs into round holes: Some comments on "An analysis of variance model for the intrasubject replication design." *Journal of Applied Behavior Analysis, 7*(4), 635–638.

Hilliard, R. B. (1993). Single-case methodology in psychotherapy process and outcome research. *Journal of Consulting and Clinical Psychology, 61*(3), 373–380.

Huck, S. W., & Cormier, W. H. (1996). *Reading statistics and research* (2nd ed.). New York: Harper Collins.

Jones, E. E. (1993). Introduction to special section: Single-case research in psychotherapy. *Journal of Consulting and Clinical Psychology, 61*(3), 371–372.

Kachigan, S. K. (1991). *Multivariate statistical analysis: A conceptual introduction* (2nd ed.). New York: Radius.

Kazdin, A. E. (1982). *Single-case research designs.* New York: Oxford University Press.

Kazdin, A. E. (1984). Statistical analyses for single-case experimental designs. In D. H. Barlow & M. Hersen (Eds.), *Single case experimental designs: Strategies for studying behavior change* (2nd ed., pp. 285–324). New York: Pergamon.

Kazdin, A. E. (1992). *Research design in clinical psychology* (3rd ed.). Needham Heights, MA: Allyn & Bacon.

Kiene, H., & von Schön-Angerer, T. (1998). Single-case causality assessment as a basis for clinical judgment. *Alternative Therapies in Health and Medicine, 4*(1), 41–47.

Lukoff, K., Edwards, D., & Miller, M. (1998). The case study as a scientific method for researching alternative therapies. *Alternative Therapies in Health and Medicine, 4*(2), 44–52.

Matsuzaki, A. (2003). *The influence of individual dance/movement therapy on self-esteem and affect expression in preschool children with a history of neglect.* Unpublished master's thesis, Drexel University, Philadelphia.

Michael, J. (1974). Statistical inference for individual organism research: Some reactions to a suggestion by Gentile, Roden, and Klein. *Journal of Applied Behavior Analysis, 7*(4), 627–628.

Morgan, D. L., & Morgan, R. K. (2001). Single-participant research design. *American Psychologist, 56*(2), 119–127.

Ruzic, A. V. (2002). *The influence of individual dance/movement therapy on the development of preschoolers in a partial psychiatric treatment program.* Unpublished master's thesis, Drexel University, Philadelphia, PA.

Spirito, A., Stark, L. J., Grace, N., & Stamoulis, D. (1991). Common problems and coping strategies reported in childhood and early adolescence. *Journal of Youth and Adolescence, 20,* 531–544.

Stake, R. (1994). Case Studies. In M. K. Denzin & Y. S. Lincoln. (Eds.), *Handbook of qualitative research* (pp. 236–247). Thousand Oaks, CA: Sage.

Stewart, N. J., McMullen, L. M., & Rubin, L. D. (1994). Movement therapy with depressed inpatients: A randomized multiple single case design. *Archives of Psychiatric Nursing, 8*(1), 22–29.

Tatum-Fairfax, A. (2003). *Dance/movement therapy impact on quality of life in clients with co-occurring HIV, addiction and mood disorders.* Unpublished master's thesis, Drexel University, Philadelphia, PA.

Tyron, W. W. (1982). A simplified time-series analysis for evaluating treatment interventions. *Journal of Applied Behavior Analysis, 15*(3), 423–429.

Vogt, P. W. (1999). *Dictionary of statistics and methodology: A nontechnical guide for the social sciences* (2nd ed.). Thousand Oaks, CA: Sage.

Ware, J., & Sherbourne, C. (1992). The MOS 36-item short-form health survey. *Medical Care, 30*(6), 473–483.

Section 3

INTERPRETIVE METHODS

AND RESEARCH CONSIDERATIONS

Chapter 7

POSTPOSITIVIST INQUIRY: MULTIPLE PERSPECTIVES AND PARADIGMS

JILL GREEN

Although I am not a dance/movement therapy researcher, my work as a dance educator constantly intersects with dance/movement therapy, and I have collaborated with a number of colleagues from the field. I do not mean to claim that each area does not have particular content and methods, nor that any dance educator can play the role of therapist. On the contrary, the integrity of each field and the expertise required to practice as dance therapist or educator should be respected and protected. However, I find myself intrigued by the number of ways theory and practice from each field can inform the other.

Interestingly, a number of arts and dance/movement therapy researchers have indicated that arts education research methods have influenced their own work. For example, Roger Grainger (1999) and Lenore Wadsworth Hervey (2000) cite Elliot Eisner, an arts education theorist, in their work and call for an aesthetically grounded "arts-based" research approach, derived from his ideas. This paradigm shift towards diverse representations of knowledge has generated ideas about how dance and the body may be used as valid forms of research, and motivates dance educators and therapists alike to seek out new alternatives to scholarly work.

Although my focus on postpositivist research in dance developed from the educational arena, the methods can be easily applied to dance/movement therapy research as well. This chapter presents a framework for postpositivist inquiry and possible applications for dance/movement therapy researchers. Additionally, I offer methods based on somatic sensitivity as part of the postpositivist approach.

POSTPOSITIVIST INQUIRY

Postpositivist inquiry is part of a new paradigm movement in research. It moves beyond what has been traditionally accepted as "good science" in regard to characteristics such as objectivity, value-free data collection and analysis, repeatability, and measurable findings. This approach provides a framework based on epistemological and ontological stances and does not reject research based on the scientific model, but rather expands the boundaries of the scholarly arena, providing methods that answer different kinds of questions: questions that are not easily or appropriately answered through statistical data, measurements, or generalizing claims.

The particular framework defining types of postpositivist inquiry discussed in this chapter is based on the work of Patti Lather (1991), an educational research and curriculum theorist, and has been discussed in my previous work (Green, 1996; Green & Stinson, 1999). This framework stresses the multiplicity of terms and meanings that describe the approach and have arisen in response to the recognition of the limitations of the positivist tradition in research. It is important to note that while the prefix *post* means "after," and the forms discussed arose after positivism, positivism should not be viewed in the past tense. To the contrary, it remains the dominant worldview for research.

Lather (1991) discusses postpositivist research in her book, *Getting Smart: Feminist Research and Pedagogy With/in the Postmodern*. She agrees with John Caputo that research is approaching a "postparadigmatic diaspora," (p. 108), a time when specific and rigid paradigms are problematic. Lather acknowledges the boundaries of the term "paradigm" but uses it as a transition toward a human science that does not neatly segregate paradigms or pose one against another (p. 107). With this in mind, Lather presented a flexibly conceived framework for postpositivist inquiry (see Table 7-I). This framework encompasses four categories: prediction, understanding, emancipation, and deconstruction. Positivism is included in this framework, as prediction. Although it differs from the three postpositivist categories in Table 7-I below, it exists along with them.

Differences Between Positivism and Postpositivism: Perspectives

The three conceptualizations that make up postpositivist research are significantly different from positivism in a number of ways. Most of these dif-

Table 7-I   POSTPOSITIVIST INQUIRY

Predict	*Understand*	*Emancipate*	*Deconstruct*
positivism	interpretive	critical	poststructural
	naturalistic	neo-Marxist	postmodern
	constructivist	feminist	post-paradigmatic
	phenomenological	praxis-oriented	diaspora
	hermeneutic	educative	
		Freirian	
		participatory	
		action research	

Note: From Lather, P. (1991). *Getting Smart: Feminist Research and Pedagogy With/in the Postmodern*, (p. 7). New York and London: Routledge.

ferences have to do with two main concepts: ontology—how we look at reality—and epistemology—how we know. Generally, positivists tend to claim that there is a real truth or a big truth that we can know. Postpositivists, on the other hand, tend to believe that reality is constructed: that we understand reality according to how we are positioned in the world in relationship to our experiences, and that our subjective positions have much to do with how we see reality and truth.[1]

Epistemologically, positivists tend to claim that we can know a "true" reality by using "objective" research methods to uncover it. In contrast, many postpositivist researchers (Denzin, 1989; Eisner, 1989; Lincoln & Guba, 1985; McLaren, 1989; Nielsen, 1990; Richardson, 1988, 1990, 1995) believe that subjectivity is not only unavoidable but may even be helpful in giving researchers and participants a meaningful understanding of people and research themes. However, socially constructed reality may not be consistent and reliable in the positivist sense, because the belief systems or stories constructed vary each time they are told. Consequently, reliability, while a basic tenet of empirical scientific research, is regarded by postpositivist researchers as a concept equally as impossible as objectivity.

Methodological Differences

The differences in perspective and approach between positivist and postpositivist approaches are reflected in methods. Positivist researchers attempt to support or refute an hypothesis, while postpositivist researchers attempt to interpret or understand a particular research context. Some postpositivist approaches (emancipatory and deconstructivist) actually strive to challenge a dominant or traditional social reality, or create change through the research process. Positivist methods strive to predict outcomes and determine measurable truths that can be generalized across contexts. Postpositivist methods usually seek out unique, multiple perspectives and meanings that are context bound.

Rather than starting with an hypothesis, postpositivist researchers tend to first ask broader questions such as "What is going on here, from the perspective of the persons having this experience? What does it mean to them? How does it come to have this meaning?" Sometimes research questions may be more specific, such as "How do students learn in a dance class?" Or for

---

[1]There are actually a number of differences within the three postpositivist categories in this respect, particularly in reference to emancipatory research. For example, Ellsworth (1992) points out that critical theorists and pedagogues tend to imbue their work with dimensions of moral and rational thought. She claims that critical theory (which focuses on social marginalization regarding areas such as race, sex, and gender) is often based on fundamental moral and political principles that are absolute. However, some critical researchers are beginning to move into the deconstructionist category where concepts such as multiple perspectives, an awareness of partial knowledge and narratives, self-reflectivity, and socially constructed realities are dominant.

dance/movement therapists, "How does a client experience his or her eating disorder?" Postpositivist researchers pursue such questions through a variety of methods including but not limited to observation, participant observation, document analysis (including artistic work), and interviewing (usually more open-ended than in traditional interviewing). Information on applying some of these methods is given in Chapter 8 (Forinash) of this volume; they allow the participant to put her/his own frame around the experience. The time required for this process, and the quantity of material generated, tends to limit the number of subjects that can be included in a study. Thus, large samples are usually not characteristic of postpositivist studies. This is not considered problematic since the findings will not be generalized to a larger population. Rather, findings are grounded in context.

Another difference between positivist and postpositivist approaches is the use and generation of theory. Positivists attempt to test theory to see if it can be supported or refuted, while postpositivist researchers generally attempt to be aware of emerging theory and create research designs to build theory through the research context. Lincoln and Guba (1985), two main proponents of what they initially termed "naturalistic inquiry," and what they later referred to as "fourth generation evaluation," claim that

> designs must be emergent because the existence of multiple realities constrains the development of a design based only on one (the investigator's) construction; because what will be learned at a site is always dependent on the interaction between the investigator and context, and the interaction is also not fully predictable; and because the nature of mutual shapings cannot be known until witnessed (p. 208).

Thus, while general procedures for data collection and analysis may provide parameters and a general guide for the study, the postpositivist researcher must remain open to emerging patterns, themes, and theories.

Data Analysis Write-up

Many postpositivist researchers argue against claims for a value-free research method (Denzin, 1989; Eisner, 1989; Fetterman, 1989; Kvale, 1983; Lather, 1986a; Guba & Lincoln, 1989; Lincoln & Guba, 1985; Maguire, 1987), and some further argue that data are not found, but rather constructed by people according to their subjectivities (Bazerman, 1987; Lather, 1991; Richardson, 1988, 1990, 1997; Van Manen, 1990; Wolcott, 1990). These postpositivists argue that the act of writing up data necessarily involves the process of interpretation, based on social constructions and the writer's preconceived assumptions about what it means to do research. Laurel Richardson (1990, 1997) claims that all writing is inscribed by our values and reflects metaphors that we use to communicate how we see the world. "Science writing" is not excluded; it uses certain conventions that express knowledge as problem centered and linear, but is displayed through a narrative form. Since writing is affected by our experiences, no data are neutral. Therefore, according to this perspective, it is effective to make one's subjectivity visible and display how one's voice as researcher enters the text. The first person voice is often used in postpositivist research in an attempt to recognize the researcher's presence and bring a sense of self-reflexivity to the process.

It is helpful to think about all research reports as a kind of storytelling. Even though most scholarly texts rely heavily on quantifiable data, they tell what John Van Maanen (1988) has named "realist tales." Realist tales employ the convention of the third person, taking the "I" out of the report in order to establish authority. Richardson (1988) has noted that when the researcher's presence is not visible, the myth of objectivity is maintained.

Although most conventional research accounts tell realist tales, there is a broad body of postpositivist literature (see Lather, 1991, 1993; Richardson, 1988, 1997) that attempts to recognize the researcher's presence and bring a sense of reflection to the process of writing up data. These accounts allow writers to reflect on their own perspectives and thus recognize how they are subjectively inscribed by their experiences and culture. They attempt to include "multiple voices" in order to display the various positions and perspectives of the researchers and participants. Often, experimental narrative forms are used as vehicles to provide a voice to those participants who may ordinarily be unheard.

The kinds of forms that may result from this process include storytelling, autobiographical accounts, split-page formats (to highlight the diverse and sometimes discrepant multiple voices), and narratives which tend to break down a particular, and usually theoretical, stance in order to disrupt the authority and assumptions of a dominant paradigm (see Lather, 1991). The presence of multiple voices may be projected through juxtapositions of art-work, dance, poetry, journal entries, and other aesthetic expressions. Artistic representations may help to display participant voices and give shape to the lived experiences of the participants (Van Manen, 1990; also see Hervey in this volume). In this way, the research becomes a kind of expressive art form, one that can be quite compatible with many questions in dance.

Validity

One final difference between positivist and postpositivist research has to with the concept of validity. Steiner Kvale (1989) provided a framework for qualitative research validity that I find particularly helpful in broad discussions about validity and trustworthiness regarding postpositivist research. Kvale claims that in qualitative research "validity concerns the justification of knowledge claims" (p. 89). Therefore, validity criteria must adequately reflect the ontological and epistemological perspectives of the research approach. Validity in positivism focuses on constructs, measurement, and the features of the research design that help to refute alternative explanations for the findings (see Berrol and Cruz & Koch in this volume), while validity in postpositivism focuses on investigation, and the generation and application of knowledge. Furthermore, since postpositivist research is not based on one conception of reality, a reliance on external validity criteria would be counterproductive, problematic, and inconsistent with the tenets of a postpositivist perspective. Because postpositivist researchers and theorists do not attempt to generalize data, they have a broader concept of validity which does not attempt to determine whether a knowledge statement corresponds to the objective world. Kvale's "coherence criterion," which refers to the "unity, consistency and internal logic of a statement," is an appropriate framework for postpositivist research (p. 75).

As a method of investigation, validation also becomes a way of checking in postpositivist research. Kvale (1989) refers to Miles and Huberman's twelve tactics for testing and confirming qualitative research findings as a way of checking sources of potential bias that may invalidate qualitative observations and interpretations. These include methods such as checking for triangulation, weighing evidence, contrasting and comparing, examining outliers, looking for negative evidence, and getting feedback from informants. According to Kvale, as a method of investigation, to validate is also to question. The researcher must continually ask what question the data are answering, and in what context. In other words, the researcher must ask "what" she or he is looking for and in what context. Although a statement may not be factually true, the researcher may be interested in the participant's perception of that truth. To question is to continually ask what is being investigated and why.

As another method of investigation, to validate is also to theorize. For Kvale validation also "leads to a theoretical and philosophical questioning of the nature of the phenomena investigated" (p. 82). He claims,

> The complexities of validating qualitative or postpositivist research need not be due to a weakness of qualitative methods, but, on the contrary, may rest upon their extraordinary power to reflect and conceptualize the nature of the phenomenon investigated, to capture the complexity of the social reality. The validation of qualitative research becomes intrinsically linked to the development of a theory of social reality (pp. 82–83).

Validity is therefore theory-related; investigating the truth of an interpretation depends upon how the researcher perceives the phenomenon studied.

Postpositivist researchers also tend to value Kvale's (1989) concept of communicative validity, or testing the validity of knowledge claims in a dialogue. This criterion requires an attempt at open communication and consensus.

In this respect, postpositivist researchers point out the need for evidence of self-reflexivity as a validity criterion. Self-reflexivity may be met through a reflective journal, which helps to sort out personal reflections and method-ological decisions as well as other reflective instruments. Kvale (1989) also calls for testing the validity of knowledge claims in dialogue through a community of scholars: Lincoln and Guba (1985) refer to this as peer debriefing; sharing data findings with colleagues who are familiar with the content of one's work as well as postpositivist methods may bring authority to the research. Outsiders may also provide feedback about methods, practices, and findings.

Finally, pragmatic validity requires that an investigation take action to pro-duce results. Lather (1986b, p. 67) refers to this as "catalytic validity." Although this might not be an appropriate criterion for interpretive approaches, it is par-ticularly significant for emancipatory approaches that seek to make societal changes or provide unconventional theoretical frameworks.

Depending on context, validity requirements change in postpositivist approaches. This is one reason why some criteria are often referred to by different names in the literature. However, there are a number of common standards used by many postpositivist researchers.

In order to illustrate validity concerns, I will provide an example from my own research. To conduct research on how students perceive their bodies in higher education dance classes, I set up a class to investigate this issue (see Green, 1999, 2000). Because I was coming from an emancipatory/liberar-tory paradigmatic stance, I addressed coherence criterion, and checked the internal logic of the context, by asking students if they experienced prob-lems with issues of body image in their dance training. Overall, they sug-gested that dance education was problematic because there was a focus on an unachievable ideal. However, I conducted member checks with the par-ticipants to see if what I was finding was indeed what they believed and expe-rienced. Additionally, I reanalyzed the data looking for discrepant cases, began to question my own assumptions, and checked reflexive statements in my field journal for disconfirming evidence. I found that one student did feel some sense of agency when working toward a bodily ideal, a response that did not fit so neatly with the rest of my findings. Through reflexive action, I found this outlier and began to question my own assumptions about the data. Although I continued to triangulate my data by bringing in new sources of data and new theories, suggesting that this sense of agency might not be real, I ended up pointing to problems with this sense of agency; reflective action and validity checks provided a richer and more complex analysis that was trustworthy in the postpositivist framework.

APPROACHES TO POSTPOSITIVIST INQUIRY AND APPLICATIONS

In this section, three different approaches to postpositivist research are discussed following Lather's (1991) conceptualization: research directed toward *understanding*, research directed toward *emancipation*, and research directed toward *deconstruction*. Possible applications are provided for each approach. It may be significant to point out that when discussing the three approaches represented in Lather's framework, the borders or boundaries of each approach are not clearly defined or static. For example, some scholars consider *critical* approaches as part of *interpretive* inquiry, while Lather generally represents it under the emancipatory heading. For purposes of clarification and discussion, I will identify these categories as separate conceptualizations so that the reader may more fully understand the characteristics of each perspective and method (see Table 7-I).

Research Directed Towards Understanding

Some subcategories under the *understanding* heading include interpretive, naturalistic, constructivist, phenomenological, and hermeneutic inquiry. These types of research are based on understanding a particular research context. The purpose is to interpret what is going on in the research setting and theorize a contextual understanding of the research problem. As in most postpositivist inquiry, the investigator does not attempt to separate her- or himself from the research context but rather recognizes the researcher's part in the study. Therefore, generally, the narrative or report of the findings embraces the subjective aspect of researcher as participant and participants as researchers. The final report of findings is constructed or built upon the data-gathering tools of the investigation.

Since the overall purpose of this category is to understand, there is a general sense of finding personal meaning. In this regard, the purpose of *interpretive* research is to create meaning by listening to the voices of the participants in the study, often including the voice of the researcher. These types of studies tend to focus on the meaning perspectives of the participants (Erickson, 1986). *Naturalistic* inquiry tends to refer to the framework created by Guba and Lincoln (1989), which strives to interpret meaning through context. In this approach, research designs emerge within the research process (Lincoln & Guba, 1985). The *constructivist* approach is similar to naturalistic and interpretive inquiry in the sense that the researcher constructs meaning and enters the research context as a participant with a particular point of view. *Phenomenological* research describes lived experience. *Hermeneutic* research is often considered part of phenomenology, as it is captured in language. It emphasizes the "interpretive dialogue between the researcher and the objects of inquiry while accepting the inevitable influences of personal, cultural and historical biases" (McNiff, 1998, p. 111).

There may be a number of applications of this *understand* category to dance/movement therapy. For example, case study research is often generated through an attempt to understand a particular context. Shaun McNiff (1998) offers some particular examples from art therapy research including exemplars from his own work, Bruce Moon's "narrative account into a new artistic dimension with his poetically written 'stories' about his experiences with his clients" (p. 64), and Debra Linesch's documentation of how "the hermeneutic approach to contextual engagement furthers the interpretation of psychotherapeutic dialogue and helps art therapists see where the imagery points rather than what meanings lie behind it" (p. 113).

Other types of research in this area may include studies that focus on the experience of particular types of therapies: not their effectiveness, but how they affect clients and/or the researcher or researcher/clinician, the relationship between the caregivers and the clients (see Grainger, 1999, p. 104), and studies that focus on the collaboration between researcher and subject, that is, where the researcher is a participant in the research (see Grainger, 1999; Hervey, 2000).

Research Directed Toward Emancipation

Although some scholars consider critical theory a part of *interpretive* research, Lather includes it in the *emancipate* category because it emphasizes what may be problematic about a particular topic and moves the researcher toward an agenda that may include social change or action. Inquiry in the emancipatory area purposely leads the researcher in a direction that addresses social and political power issues that emerge from the research. The emancipatory researcher brings a critical perspective, one that may include issues such as race, gender, class, sexuality, et cetera. Often, the investigation is part of a social advocacy project, and there is an attempt to change participants and society.

Critical research reflects critical social theory and generally calls for social and economic justice. It rejects inequality, the oppression of disenfranchised groups, the silencing of marginalized voices, and authoritarian social structures and institutions. *Neo-Marxist* research emphasizes economics and attempts to shift power to a minority (Bell, 1980).

Additionally, Daniel Bell (1980) suggests that neo-Marxism no longer address the socialist ideas of Marxism but embraces the idea of "alienation in its stead" (p. 184). Thus while critical theory as a whole addresses issues of the disenfranchised in a number of areas, such as race, class, and gender, neo-Marxism is more specifically rooted in classicism, yet, no longer addresses a socialist framework.

Feminist research focuses on issues of gender, although many feminists today have developed research agendas that critique other issues as well. It is significant to note that there are many types of feminism. These approaches stress women's marginal status in society and culture, and include other disenfranchised peoples as social groupings.

Praxis-oriented, Freirian, participatory, and *action research* are terms associated with Paulo Freire, a Brazilian educator and theorist who critiqued the educational system and called for a move towards equality and justice (Leach, 1982). They represent approaches that embrace practice and action: complex activities by which individuals become critically social conscious humans.

Participatory research aims for social change and challenges the way knowledge is both produced and disseminated via conventional social science methods and dominant educational institutions. Using alternative methods, participatory research attempts to put the production of knowledge into the hands of the people so that struggles for social equality and the elimination of dependency and its symptoms (for example, poverty, illiteracy, and malnutrition) can be empowered.

In dance education and some dance/movement therapy settings, this type of research can refer to the participation of both researcher and participants in all aspects of a study. For example, it can mean that the participants help design or analyze the data, or that the researcher is a participant, such as if a dance educator researcher takes a class she or he is researching or a dance/movement therapy researcher becomes a participant in a therapeutic program.

Action research is related to participatory research; some scholars use the terms interchangeably. However, it is significant to point out that the term, action research, has been used in different ways by diverse scholars and researchers. Lather (1991) points to an emphasis on social action related to the term, and this is why she includes it under the *emancipate* category. The point is to engage the participants in the study but there is a further goal: to create social change.

A number of educational and creative arts therapy researchers have used action research in a more practical, participatory way that has included viewing participants in a social context that has not extended to the goal of social change. For example, Grainger (1999) discusses action research much like participatory research and emphasizes interaction rather than social change. He posits that action research involves the use of as many sources of information as possible. Instead of concentrating on observations registered by an observer presumed by his or her scientific attitude of mind to be detached, this approach "concerns itself directly with the experience of everyone involved, both as investigator and investigated" (pp. 99–100).

McNiff (1998) and a number of other arts therapy and education researchers conceptualize action research in relationship to change but change within a particular context, rather than social change. McNiff states that action research "uses the investigation as a way of encouraging change within a particular setting" (p. 113). Recently, action research has been used exclusively in this way by a number of therapists and researchers. In the educational arena, action research has often signified the practice of researching one's own teaching and reflecting on it in order to create effective pedagogical changes in particular courses.

For the reasons discussed above, these types of frameworks for action research would be more appropriate for the *understand* category than the *emancipatory* category in Lather's (1991) conceptualization, since they do not always have a primary goal of social change. Lather's definition of action research is a better fit for the emancipatory category.

There are a number of applications of the *emancipatory* category. Much of my work falls into this category. For example, I investigated how students have been traditionally taught in higher education dance, and looked at issues such as power and authority in dance classes, particularly in reference to body image ideals and how dance students are expected to behave in dance class (see Green, 1999, 2000, 2001a, 2001b).

This type of research may be applied to dance/movement therapy in a number of ways. For example, dance/movement therapy researchers might investigate how particular therapy practices may or may not help clients in the long run. They might look into practices that may be interpreted by their clients as oppressive rather than liberating. Dance/movement therapists might also question particular therapeutic relationships and use their research to call for practices that are more egalitarian or liberating than standard practices. They might also study the costs of dance/movement therapy, and its accessibility to various marginalized groups, or how as a westernized practice, it may not fully reach peoples of particular cultures.

Research Directed Towards Deconstruction

Deconstructive research is not really a method, but more of a way of thinking (Lather, 1991) often embodied through a literary form that reflects postmodern thought. Postmodernism can be conceptualized in a number of ways. Some scholars refer to a post-foundational postmodern perspective that challenges theories that are reliant on the concept of universal truths; others speak more generally of living in a postmodern world of conflicting and competing ideas and worldviews. In other words, postmodernism may be thought of as a state of the world in which diverse ideas bump up against each other, or as a theoretical perspective itself. Lather's (1991) framework as a whole projects a sense of postmodern multiplicity, while the *deconstructivist* category specifically reflects postmodern thought.

Parpart (1992) summarizes the main themes of postmodern thought through a discussion of such postmodernists as Lyotard, Foucault, and Derrida. Basically, she claims that postmodern thinkers have questioned assumptions of the modern age such as the belief that reason and scientific inquiry can provide an objective and universal foundation for knowledge. Thus, postmodernism professes a view that challenges assumptions of universal and dominant meaning systems. While postmodernism addresses this particular view, deconstructivist and postmodern research primarily demonstrate particular writing practices. These discursive practices display privileged discourses and multiple realities through narrative literary forms that include: a) split page formats, where the voices of participants, for example, may be typed on one side, while the voice of the researcher is typed on the other side in order to display the multiple and sometimes discrepant ideas that came from the research; b) the use of various types of fonts to connote diverse perspectives; c) artwork; and d) other narrative forms. Often the silenced voices of marginalized and disenfranchised groups are juxtaposed against the researcher's authoritative voice (see Lather, 1991; and Green, 1993, for examples of deconstructivist stories). All realities, including the author's written account, are admittedly partial and problematic. According to Lather (1991), the goal of deconstruction "is neither unitary wholeness nor dialectical resolution. The goal of deconstruction is to keep things in process, to disrupt, to keep the system in play, to set up procedures to continuously demystify the realities we create, and to fight the tendency for our categories to congeal" (p. 13).

The deconstructivist researcher seeks ways to display multiple realities; as Lather (1991) notes, this is done "in order to juxtapose alternative representations and foreground the very constructed nature of our knowing" (p. 136). Even the concept of lived experience, so prominent in interpretive research, is viewed as a construction dependent on who is doing the experiencing. Although some interpretive and emancipatory research may ultimately deconstruct dominant meaning systems, this is not usually the primary intent. However, this example points out the problematic nature of the multiple categories that have been created for postpositivist research.

There are a number of examples of how deconstructivist research may be applied to dance/movement therapy. The researcher might highlight, for example, how a therapist's training and communication style reflect attitudes constructed through the history of dance and clinical psychology. The researcher might observe how the therapist perceives her or his role as authority figure, perhaps by purporting to "know what is best" for the client. The researcher might look at the therapist's own background and training as well as the influence of traditional dance/movement therapy training on her or his own style. Finally, the researcher might provide an historical deconstruction or historical analysis of power in dance/movement therapy training in the form of a series of case studies of dance therapists.

SOMATIC SENSITIVITY AS A POSTPOSITIVIST RESEARCH TOOL

Postpositivist inquiry, particularly the emancipatory and deconstructive categories, calls for self reflexivity and the multiple, expressive voices of the participants and researcher(s). Since the dancing body is the content of the work in dance/movement therapy, somatic sensitivity may be an appropriate tool for self reflection in this field. Reflective body awareness may enable researchers to read the research from another (physical) perspective, "decenter" uncritical assumptions about a particular research context, and question their own beliefs. In this sense, somatic practice and sensitivity may resonate with a "postmodern turn" away from a clear certainty or single truth. It embraces multiple positions, diverse perspectives, and an inner physical struggle with emerging ideas and issues (see Green, 1994).

There are a number of ways to emphasize somatic sensitivity throughout a study. Researchers may, for example, include somatic practice during an ongoing investigation. While working with students on research projects, I often take time out to focus on the body and include experiential somatic work as a way of allowing students to express how they are dealing with the issues raised in the study (see Green, 1993, 1994, 1999, 2000, 2001a, 2001b). After discussing critical problems associated with media and body image, students are allowed time to focus on body awareness in order to see how they perceived the material and how their own bodies were affected by the discussion and issues it raised.

Additionally, as a researcher, I have attempted to pay attention to bodily signals such as a faster beating heart, sweaty palms, et cetera, in an attempt to read my own take on what was happening during the research project and how I was responding to, for instance, comments made by the participants or their resistance to the work. Further, I have looked at my somatic responses as both teacher and researcher in participant studies, to evaluate how my particular roles were affecting the research. Dance/movement therapy researchers may similarly note these types of experiences and sensations while participating in the therapy process as well as the research process.

Moreover, dance/movement therapy researchers might reflect on a bodily basis by engaging in a somatic reading of a particular topic, context, or theory. For example, during a literature review, a researcher may take note of bodily sensation regarding diverse theoretical perspectives and views, particularly while doing deconstructive research when many theories and viewpoints may bump up against each other. Somatic tensions may be revealed within the narrative story along with other findings. In my own research, after wrestling with a particularly difficult body of literature I noted,

> After much review of literature in feminism and postmodernism, my body began to communicate disturbing messages as I struggled with the material. My state of ease and bliss was shaken. After reading about the possibility of social construction and a foundationalism tied to modernist and humanistic texts, I began to look back at what I had written with a certain queasiness. I began to cringe and feel my skin crawl as I reread some of my writings, specifically sections on creativity, as I became acutely aware of how my initial positioning was reflected in the text. I noticed that I universalized meaning without reference to a social context and defined creativity by assumed universal attributes. I also was aware that initially I had done the same with somatics, limiting it to an individualistic context alone. Rereading my own text from

a postmodern perspective, all the big "Truths" popped out at me as I experienced a painful questioning of everything I had previously been so confident about; I felt an existential angst on a very profound level and somatically, I began to feel a postmodern turn[ing] of my stomach as I realized the literatures do not necessarily come together neatly (Green, 1994, p. 13).

CLOSING THOUGHTS

It makes sense that dance/movement therapy researchers use tools that are appropriate for creative arts modalities and aesthetic ways of knowing the world. Postpositivist research and bodily practices may offer effective frameworks and methods for those researchers involved in the creative arts therapies. Educational models, such as Lather's (1991) postpositivist framework, may further help dance/movement therapy researchers find methodologies that resonate with the theories and practices inherent in the field.

It should be apparent from the description in this chapter that postpositivist research is not a monolith. Postpositivist researchers have disagreements with each other and the many categories of this type of research are not firmly fixed. New forms are continually emerging. However, this may be something that dance/movement therapists can embrace since creativity is so inherent in the practice and the research process; methodologies may change and emerge throughout the investigation. Two of the reasons I am so drawn to this type of research are its creative possibilities as well as its fluid process. In this sense, postpositivist research may be thought of as an artistic process because its categories are flexible, and researchers and participants may be multi-positioned and move fluidly and creatively throughout the framework. Additionally, in seeking multiple and diverse perspectives, writing the results of a postpositivist project can be a creative process itself. Postpositivist research allows for the juxtaposition of data and findings through an artistic pastiche of diverse voices and perspectives. These multiple and moving views reflect the ontology, epistemology, and creative possibilities of postmodernism itself.

REFERENCES

Bazerman, C. (1987). The APA publication manual as a behaviorist rhetoric. In J. Nelson, A. Megill, & D. N. McCloskley (Eds.), *The rhetoric of the human sciences* (pp. 125–144). Madison, WI: University of Wisconsin Press.

Bell, D. (1980). The social sciences since the second world war–Part two. In M. Adler (Ed.), *The great ideas today* (pp. 184–232). Chicago, IL: Encyclopedia Britannica.

Denzin, N. K. (1989). *The research act: A theoretical introduction to sociological methods* (3rd ed.). Englewood Cliffs, NJ: Prentice Hall.

Eisner, E. (1989). Objectivity and subjectivity in qualitative research and evaluation. In E. W. Eisner & A. M. Peshkin (Eds.), *Qualitative studies in education.* New York: Teachers College Press.

Ellsworth, E. (1992). Why doesn't this feel empowering? Working through the repressive myths of critical pedagogy. In C. Luke & J. Gore (Eds.), *Feminism and critical pedagogy* (pp. 90–119). New York: Routledge.

Erickson, F. (1986). Qualitative methods in research on teaching. In M. C. Wittrock (Ed.), *Handbook of research on teaching* (3rd ed., pp. 119–161). New York: Macmillan.

Fetterman, D. M. (1989). *Ethnography step by step.* Newbury Park, CA: Sage.

Grainger, R. (1999). *Researching the arts therapies: Dramatherapist's perspective.* London and Philadelphia: Jessica Kingsley.

Green, J. (1993). Fostering creativity through movement and body awareness practices: A postpositivist investigation into the relationship between somatics and the creative process (Doctoral dissertation, The Ohio State University, 1993). Dissertation Abstracts International, 54 (11), 3910A.

Green, J. (1994). *A postmodern turn[ing] of the stomach: Somatic sensitivity as a qualitative research tool.* Unpublished manuscript.

Green, J. (1996). Moving through and against multiple paradigms: postpositivist research in somatics and creativity–Part I. *Journal of Interdisciplinary Research in Physical Education, 1*(1), 43–54.

Green, J. (1999). Somatic authority and the myth of the ideal body in dance education. *Dance Research Journal, 31*(2), 80–100.

Green, J. (2000). Socially constructed bodies in American dance classrooms. *Research in Dance Education, 2*(2),155–173.

Green, J. (2001a). Emancipatory pedagogy? Women's bodies and the creative process in dance. *Frontiers: A Journal of Women's Studies, 21*(3), 124–140.

Green, J. (2001b). Social somatic theory, practice, and research: An inclusive approach in higher education. *Conference Proceedings, Dancing in the Millennium: An International Conference* (pp. 213–217). Washington, D.C.

Green, J., & Stinson, S.W. (1999). Postpositivist research in dance. In S. H. Fraleigh & P. Hanstein (Eds.) *Researching dance: Evolving modes of inquiry* (pp. 91–123). Pittsburgh, PA: University of Pittsburgh Press.

Guba, E., & Lincoln, Y. S. (1989). *Fourth generation evaluation.* Newbury Park, CA: Sage.

Hervey, L. W. (2000). *Artistic inquiry in dance movement therapy: Creative alternatives for research.* Springfield, IL: Charles C Thomas.

Kvale, S. (1983). The qualitative research interview: A phenomenological and hermeneutical mode of understanding. *Journal of Phenomenological Psychology, 14,* 171–196.

Kvale, S. (1989). To validate is to question. In S. Kvale (Ed.), *Issues of validity in qualitative research* (pp. 73–92). Sweden: Student Literature.

Lather, P. (1986a). Research as praxis. *Harvard Educational Review, 56*(3), 257–277.

Lather, P. (1986b). Issues of validity in openly ideological research: Between a rock and a soft place. *Interchange, 17*(4), 63–84.

Lather, P. (1991). *Getting smart: Feminist research and pedagogy with/in the postmodern.* New York: Routledge.

Lather, P. (1993). Fertile obsession: Validity after poststructuralism. *The Sociological Quarterly, 34*(4), 673–693.

Leach, T. (1982). Paulo Freire: Dialogue, politics and relevance. *International Journal of Lifelong Education, 1*(3), 185–201.

Lincoln, Y. S., & Guba, E. (1985). *Naturalistic inquiry.* Beverly Hills, CA: Sage.

Maguire, P. (1987). *Doing participatory research: A feminist approach.* Amherst, MA: Center for International Education.

McLaren, P. (1989). *Life in schools: An introduction to critical pedagogy in the foundations of education.* New York: Longman.

McNiff, S. (1998). *Art-based research.* London and Philadelphia: Jessica Kingsley.

Nielsen ,J. M. (1990). Introduction. In J. M. Nielsen (Ed.), *Feminist research methods: Exemplary readings in the social sciences* (pp. 1–37). Boulder, CO: Westview.

Parpart, J. L. (1992). *Who is the "other?" A postmodern critique of women and development theory and practice.* Unpublished manuscript.

Richardson, L. (1988). The collective story: Postmodernism and the writing of sociology. *Sociological Focus, 21*(3), 199–208.

Richardson, L. (1990). *Writing strategies: Reaching diverse audiences* (Qualitative Research Methods Series 21). Newbury Park, CA: Sage.

Richardson, L. (1995). Writing stories: Co-authoring "The Sea Monster," a writing story. *Qualitative Inquiry, 1*(2), 189–203.

Richardson, L. (1997). *Fields of play: Constructing an academic life.* New Brunswick, NJ: Rutgers University Press.

Van Maanen, J. (1988). *Tales of the field.* Chicago, IL: University of Chicago Press.

Van Manen, M. (1990). *Researching lived experience: Human science for an action sensitive pedagogy.* Albany, NY: State University of New York Press.

Wolcott, H. (1990). *Writing up qualitative research* (Qualitative Research Methods Series 20). Newbury Park, CA: Sage.

Chapter 8

QUALITATIVE DATA COLLECTION AND ANALYSIS: INTERVIEWS, OBSERVATIONS, AND CONTENT ANALYSIS

MICHELE FORINASH

In the past ten years qualitative research has been extensively applied in the various creative arts therapies (Aigen, 1993, 1996, 1997, 1998; Blumenefeld-Jones, 1995; Bruscia, 1995; Forinash, 1993; Forinash & Lee, 1998; Hervey, 2000; Higgens, 2000; McNiff, 1998; Reynolds, 2000; Wheeler, 1995). This natural fit of qualitative research to the practice of the creative arts therapies, and dance/movement therapy in particular, is quite easy to understand when one looks at the commonalties between the two.

Aigen (1993) articulates these common ideas that are embraced by both therapy, especially humanistic approaches, and qualitative research. First he mentions *the researcher as instrument.* This means that individuals function as a real people in both the role of therapist and in the role of researcher. Humanness is a necessary tool one must have in order to relate to and engage clients, and qualitative researchers find that humanness is the best tool to understand human experiences. Aigen discusses having clients or consumers rather than patients in therapy. In qualitative research this translates into having research participants rather than research subjects. The words "participant" and "client" imply that they have an active role in the process. Underscoring this fact, the *Publication Manual of the American Psychological Association* (American Psychological Association, 2001) no longer allows the use of "subjects" when referring to research participants.

Another area Aigen (1993) discusses is *transformation.* Therapists are often transformed by experiences with clients that help them continue to grow and change. Qualitative researchers are also deeply impacted by their research endeavors and the deepening understanding they gain as they study the diversity of human experience. *Trust* is also significant in both relationships. Therapists know that therapy cannot proceed until they have established trust and rapport with their clients. In qualitative research trust between researcher and participant is equally important for meaningful results to be found.

Aigen (1993) next discusses the *stance of the researcher.* Therapists constantly seek supervision to keep their own biases and values in check. In

125

qualitative research, peers are used to help researchers debrief and recognize and articulate their worldview and assumptions that impact the ability to be present with data.

The theme of *generalizability* also bears on both relationships. In therapy, the uniqueness of the individual is valued and one is less interested in generalizing one individual's journey in therapy to others. Similarly, in qualitative research one is interested in providing a profound understanding of a specific phenomenon or event rather than providing predictions regarding future encounters.

Aigen (1993) also discusses the necessity of having a *flexible research approach*. Flexibility is valued by therapists, who recognize that therapy often takes unexpected twists and turns, and the therapist must be prepared to move with these changes. In qualitative research, open-ended research methods unfold as phenomena are engaged and examined and the researcher lets the unfolding process of the research guide him or her.

ONTOLOGY, EPISTEMOLOGY, AND METHODOLOGY

In previous publications there was a tendency to break research into two distinct categories—quantitative as compared to qualitative, also known as "positivist" versus "naturalist" (Aigen, 1991; Wheeler, 1995). As positivism developed refinements (e.g., logical positivism, falsification, and confirmation) over time, also more recently, authors have begun to further examine naturalist categories and have created additional divisions. They begin with a discussion of world view.

All research emanates from a world view—a belief of how the world functions that is referred to as *ontology*. Basing her research on that of Guba (1990) and Guba and Lincoln (1994), Edwards (1999) identifies four possible ontological positions from which to choose. The first is positivism, which states that absolute truth exists and it can be discovered: that "natural order exists outside of individual experience of events or phenomena" (Edwards, 1999, p. 75). In other words, this view holds that there is an objective reality that can be known through research; that the world is ultimately knowable and predictable.

The second position is *postpositivism*, which holds that there is an absolute and knowable reality, but the researcher's focus defines the dimensions of "the 'truth' which can be revealed through investigation. Multiple perspectives or methods are required to glimpse or approximate the truth of an experience" (Edwards, 1999, p. 75). In other words, through a variety of research methods we can gain a probable or relative truth.

The third position is *constructivism*, which states that there is no absolute reality. Rather, reality is constructed by those experiencing it. It is not important to pursue a "truth." What is important is examining how individuals construct reality through experiences that they share with others.

The final position is *critical theory*. This position holds that research questions are "derived from the social context in which values are constructed and enforced" (Edwards, 1999, p. 75). In other words all research questions emanate from a social context that allows those in positions of power in the culture to pursue research questions. Thus, this position holds that the research questions that have been asked thus far have been determined by those who hold power in the social context.

Once we have determined our ontological position, we then move to a discussion of the types of research questions we ask and the types of information or knowledge that satisfy these questions. We refer to this as our *epistemology*. If we come from a postpositivist position we might ask "Was dance movement therapy effective for a *specific* group of adolescent girls with eating disorders?" believing that we might be able to locate or identify a "truth" for this particular group of girls. If we come from a constructivist ontology we might ask "What do children in medical settings experience in dance/movement therapy and what meaning does it offer them?" believing that understanding their personal, individual experiences will shed light on the phenomenon of dance/movement therapy. If we begin from a critical theory ontology we might ask "How have our ideas and values about the role of the traditional medical community been shaped by the culture of power, and how has that impacted the field of dance/movement therapy?" believing that society's faith in the medical community is a result of the social context.

Having now identified our research questions, we next address *methods*. It can become more complex at this level because some—but not all—of the research methods discussed below can be used in more than one of the ontological positions mentioned above. Qualitative research is still developing and consequently is not a static or completely defined field. Different researchers often offer different definitions for the various research methods they use. Thus the burden often lies upon the reader to carefully examine any given article to determine the ontological position of the researcher and how it impacts the research methods. That being said, we now examine general research methods and techniques most often used under the heading of qualitative research.

Heuristic Research

Heuristic research is the study of one's personal experience (Moustakes, 1990). Moustakes first articulated the use of heuristic research as he studied his own experience of loneliness (1961, 1972, 1975). Moustakes (1990) articulated the stages in heuristic research. The first stage is *engagement*. Most clinicians who are reflective in their practices have engaged with, or thought about, an idea or a question for some time. Heuristic research questions are not born overnight, but come forth after multiple experiences that leave us with unanswered questions. Once a research question is articulated, the researcher moves into the *immersion stage*. As it implies, in this stage the researcher lives, eats, and breathes the question. It will often turn up in dreams or suddenly be seen everywhere. In the third stage, that of *incubation*, the researcher often takes a step back from the question. This is a time of inwardly nurturing all the information that has been gathered in the immersion stage. The fourth stage is *illumination*. This is the inspirational or "aha" moment, where new understandings of the data and the research question become conscious. *Explication* follows: this is where the researcher moves beyond the transformative moment and returns to the data to further study and analyze it and make sense of it in a new and more profound way. This stage entails the hard work (perspiration) required to fully examine the new meanings uncovered. *Creative synthesis* is the final stage, and while often the most difficult stage for a novice researcher, this is the stage in which the researcher takes the knowledge gleaned about personal experience and re-contextualizes it in terms of the current knowledge in the field. One's inner experience now has meaning to others—either in helping others to understand their experiences more deeply or in articulating previously unarticulated questions in the field.

Ethnographic Research

Ethnographic research is "a description and interpretation of a cultural or social group or system" (Creswell, 1998, p. 58). This differs from the case study as presented by Chaiklin and Chaiklin in this text in purpose and the degree of immersion of the researcher in the cultural or social group or system as a participant-observer. For more information on ethnography, see the chapter by Hanna in this text on anthropological methods. Often ethnographers will study cultural groups such as a particular unit in a hospital, or an inclusion classroom integrating dance/movement therapy, or a day treatment facility for adults with mental illness. Researchers pay special attention to the group's behaviors and customs.

While there is no set protocol for this style of research, the researcher generally functions as a participant-observer in the culture and becomes immersed in the activities of the culture.

Spaniol's study (1998) provides an excellent example of ethnographic research. She studied the culture of art therapy consumers who had psychiatric disabilities. She began by finding a *gatekeeper*—someone who could help her gain access to the consumers. Once she had interviewed one consumer, she asked for his help in identifying other consumers who would be interested in participating in the study. She continued interviewing consumers until she felt she had a good understanding of the culture. Through her data analysis (see the later section in this chapter) she then began to develop composite descriptions of the consumers and of their experiences in art therapy. Her findings were surprising in that she found that the art therapy consumers often wanted art therapists to focus more on the product of the art therapy sessions and not just focus on the process of the sessions. In addition she found that clients wanted fewer directives and more choices regarding the art-making process and wanted to have art as a "natural extension of people's everyday lives" (p. 35). These findings obviously have implications for dance/movement therapy. Dance/movement therapists might want to do research to find out if dance/movement therapy clients would appreciate a focus on technique in addition to process and less focus on directives, and how clients might integrate dance into their lives outside of the therapy session.

Grounded Theory Research

Grounded theory is a research method which seeks to generate theory that relates to particular experiences (Creswell, 1998, p. 56). In other words, the researcher does an in-depth study of a phenomenon or event and then generates a theory which explains or describes the phenomenon or event. Creswell writes that the researcher does interviews with those engaged in the phenomenon until the researcher is *saturated* or unable to find any new information on the phenomenon. Interviews are then analyzed in a systematic manner which includes *open coding, axial coding, selective coding,* and then the development of a *conditional matrix* (p. 57).

While it is beyond the scope of this chapter to discuss this method in depth, an excellent example can be found in a study by Amir (1996). She studied both music therapists and music therapy clients to "illuminate how meaningful moments in the music therapy process were experienced by both therapists and clients" (p. 111). Through extensive interviewing and analysis she offers theory regarding the "general characteristics of meaningful moments" (p. 119). This includes essential aspects such as spontaneity, ineffability, and multiplicity of experience. She goes on to articulate types of meaningful moments that occurred in the music therapy process including moments of awareness and insight, acceptance, freedom, wholeness, completion, beauty, spirituality, intimacy, ecstasy, anger, surprise, and transformation. She also provides theory for the environmental factors and intrapersonal factors which allowed these moments to emerge.

Trustworthiness in Qualitative Research

As can be seen in the previous discussion, there are many qualitative methods that do not follow specific protocols, but instead follow the unfolding of the phenomenon as it presents itself. This leads to questions of how one can establish validity and trustworthiness in this type of research.

Various writers have been articulating approaches to address issues of trustworthiness. Bruscia (1998) presents four general areas of *integrity* with which to evaluate research. He states that these areas are not to be used as a checklist per se, but rather these areas help both the researcher and the reader evaluate the study: "The standards set forth here are constructs of the author which are intended for application only where relevant to the phenomenon, participants, and lived worlds under inquiry by the researcher. They are not meant to be universal or consensual" (p. 182).

The first area he defines is that of *methodological integrity*, for which he proposes these guidelines. The method should be both flexible and appropriate to the topic being studied. There should be an ongoing relationship with the participants that is also known as prolonged engagement (Lincoln & Guba, 1985) to ensure meaningful results. There should be persistent observation, which refers to the researcher's continual examination of the research question.

The next area Bruscia (1998) defines is that of *personal integrity*. This refers to the "Values a researcher follows when defining his/her role, responsibilities and identity in relation to the study" (p. 189). His guidelines for personal integrity are authenticity and caring. Authenticity refers to the researchers striving "to be fully who they are within the context of the research both personally and professionally" (p. 190). This includes having a serious intent, staying open to new findings, taking responsibility for one's methodological steps, and communicating clearly with all those involved in the study.

Interpersonal integrity, the third area Bruscia defines, refers to the values "the researcher demonstrates when relating to all involved in the study" (1998, p. 185). The guidelines for this area include the researcher's attempt to understand the participants in their cultural and personal worlds; checking his/her observations and interpretations with the participants in the study; and the researcher using a peer group to debrief and discuss how the researcher's personal values and biases are impacting the study. This area also refers to the researcher respecting and honoring the rights of each individual.

Finally Bruscia (1998) defines *aesthetic integrity*, which refers to the qualities of beauty in the study. While at first this may seem unusual, when one reflects on the practice of dance/movement therapy and the other arts therapies, one realizes that much of the theoretical base is built on the idea of aesthetics. Hence the research methods should also demonstrate this level of integrity. Bruscia refers to the relevance of the study, the creativity of the study, and the new awareness brought forth in the study as guidelines for aesthetic integrity.

Stige (2002) provides a different lens through which to view issues of evaluation and trustworthiness in qualitative research. Using the acronym "ERIC" he defines four general areas of concern.

E—refers to the relevance and solidity of *empirical materials*. Stige defines this as the integrity and completeness of all field notes, observations, audio/video recordings, and interviews. These materials must not be arbitrary and fragmented but rather complete, demonstrating a prolonged engagement and persistent observation with the phenomenon under study (Lincoln & Guba, 1985).

R—refers to the problem of *representation*. Stige defines this as the unique problem we face as researchers in the creative arts therapies. Any use of language to portray our experience involves a distortion of the phenomenon. In writing about experiences in the creative arts therapies one is translating into words what occurred in a different realm. A literal translation can often miss the essence of the experience. This served as the starting point for artistic inquiry or the arts-based research methods addressed in this text by Hervey (see Chapter 11). Hence the researcher must be aware and responsive to the problems of language.

I—refers to *interpretation*. Stige defines this as the biases and pre-understandings the researcher brings to the research endeavor. Even choosing the research question and how to collect the data is influenced by the researcher's beliefs and world view. Thus the researcher must have an awareness of his/her own biases and through various constructs such as triangulation, peer debriefing, and member checks (Lincoln & Guba, 1985), both acknowledge those biases and work through them as much as possible.

C—refers to the social and political *context* in which the research is situated. The context influences the types of research questions that are asked. Stige's definition includes the researcher's responsibility not to let the research contribute to repression and disempowerment. As dance/movement therapists and other creative arts therapists often work with individuals who are marginalized by society, it is especially important that they focus on empowering others through research.

Stige (2002) ends by discussing a general need for *reflexivity*—a willingness to thoroughly examine and question all aspects of research endeavors. This reflexivity, which is a hallmark of clinical practice, finds an equally important place in research.

As the various research methods can differ greatly in qualitative research, there is no checklist that lets researchers determine credibility and trustworthiness. Rather, they must adopt a mind-set with a general awareness of the issues that one must consider when pursuing research.

Interviewing and Observing

Often in qualitative research, researchers use interviewing and observing as ways of collecting data. Researchers trained in dance/movement therapy or other modalities have often developed some of the necessary skills for interviewing and observing in their training as clinicians.

Janesick (1998) defines interviewing as "a meeting of two persons to exchange information and ideas through questions and responses, resulting in communication and joint construction of meaning about a particular topic" (p. 30). She provides specific guidelines for interviewing such as preparedness and courtesy. Preparedness includes assembling materials ahead of time including a working tape recorder, a notebook for recording field-notes, and extra batteries and tapes. Issues of courtesy involve such things as ending on time, thanking the interviewee, and being respectful regarding the privacy of the interviewee.

Janesick (1998) identifies specific types of questions used in interviews. I have found this very useful in teaching students the art of interviewing. She begins with *basic descriptive questions* which are open-ended, asking for both a reporting of events and feelings. This allows the researcher to get an overall sense of the interviewee's experience, yet it is important that the researcher not let this open-ended question become the only question asked in the interview! A researcher might ask "Can you tell me about being a dance therapist with children with autism? Can you describe how you are feeling when you do the work?" *Follow-up questions* are those that the researcher uses to further clarify something the interviewee had previously mentioned. A researcher might ask "You mentioned that you felt dance therapy provided a safety valve for these children—can you say more about that?" *Example questions* ask the interviewee to provide an example of a concept previously mentioned. The researcher might ask "Can you give me an example of a time when you were really engaged with a child in a session-what were you doing and how did you feel?"

Clarification questions are those which ask the interviewee to define or clarify the meaning of a topic that has been mentioned. A researcher might ask "You have mentioned 'holding environment' several times—can you clarify what that term means to you?" *Paradigmatic questions* help the researcher understand the interviewee's basic underlying beliefs. These are questions such as "What are your core beliefs about dance movement therapy with children with autism? What keeps you engaged in what some might see as a challenging area of practice?" *Comparison questions* ask the interviewee to describe the differences between a set of experiences. A researcher might ask "You have mentioned being very active in a session and at other times being much less active. Can you describe the differences between those experiences?" (Janesick, 1998, pp. 30–31). I would add to this list *closing questions* which allow the interviewee to add any comments or discuss something the researcher may not have asked, but that the interviewee feels is important.

Observing is especially important in the creative arts therapies as one is interested in studying not only verbal participation but also nonverbal participation. Dance/movement therapy has many different theoretical orientations by which to observe or analyze movement (Bartenieff, Davis, & Paulay, 1970; Laban & Lawrence, 1947; Laban, 1960; Lewis & Loman, 1990; Sandel, Chaiklin, & Lohn, 1993), which can easily be included in research.

Janesick (1998) also discusses observation. She cites an early dance teacher who asked her class to observe her carefully so that the students could become deeply aware of their bodies and minds and "internalize the movement" (p. 13). This is perhaps the key to observing—to look so fully and deeply that one has a felt sense of what one is seeing. Other relevant aspects of movement observation for dance/movement therapists are addressed by Cruz and Koch in this volume (see Chapter 4).

It is very useful as a researcher to begin to analyze one's typical way of observing. Janesick (1998) advises that researchers, through a series of tasks, become aware of their inherent biases when approaching observation. One exercise is to observe objects on a table from multiple places in the room. In each location the student should describe what is seen as completely as possible. In comparing notes with other students in the room, one can quickly become aware of what parts of the experience one tends to focus on and what parts one tends to take for granted.

Janesick (1998) also stresses that students need to develop a system of coding their observations. This includes not only the observations, but also personal feelings and experiences that arise in the process of observing. She takes it one step further in asking that students do a self evaluation after each observation exercise, citing what they learned about themselves, what they need to work on to improve their observation skills, and a description of how they are progressing in the observational skills.

How to Analyze Data

Regardless of which qualitative method one chooses to use, one will undoubtedly at some point have amassed a mountain of data. Whether it is in the form of interview transcripts, videotapes, artifacts, or art projects, as a researcher one has to ask oneself what to do with it all.

There are many ways of analyzing data. It is important to remember that there is no one way to do it correctly. However, a useful outline is devising a plan for analysis, testing it out to see if it is useful, and revising the plan for analysis.

What follows is a general protocol that many researchers use for analyzing data. It can be modified and changed as needed. It is adapted from the method by Giorgi (1984). There are two general areas in the analysis. The first is the deconstruction of the data. Once the data are thoroughly deconstructed and understood, the researcher then reconstructs the data and, in this process, uncovers new meanings and awareness of the phenomenon.

In deconstruction, the first step is to take the data and review them in their entirety. For transcripts and videotapes this means reading through or watching them and jotting down ideas that come up while reading or viewing. For art projects or artifacts, it means examining them and recording any thoughts, feelings, or observations.

The second step is to again review the data, only more slowly and in-depth, with the idea of focusing on the data as they are presented. The researcher can highlight quotes from the interviews or make notes based on observations of the data. In this step staying open to new awareness is important, as is allowing oneself to be present in a meaningful way with the data. It is often easy and tempting to jump to quick conclusions at this stage, because living in the temporary uncertainty of the data is quite daunting. It may be that this step includes multiple reviews of the data—perhaps at different times of the day or in different frames of mind—all to ensure the most thorough analysis possible. A peer research support group can help provide a researcher with feedback regarding the depth of the review of the data.

When the researcher feels truly saturated with the data it is time to move to the next step. In this step the researcher begins to form categories, meaning units, or themes based on the material that was highlighted or observed in the previous step. Again these themes will not fall perfectly into place, but with time, persistence, and negotiating with the data, it will begin to make sense. It is at this stage that beginning researchers often feel frustrated. There is no one correct way to organize the themes. It takes trial and error, willingness to "not know," and an immersion in the data before it can really come together.

Based on an understanding of the various themes that have emerged, the researcher now reconstructs the experience. He or she provides a thorough description of the phenomenon being studied, discussing both the essential structures as well as the individual or unique aspects of the phenomenon. This reconstruction should yield new information, new perspectives, new awareness, or some enlightened view of the phenomenon. Again the peer research support group can serve to provide feedback to the researcher regarding the thoroughness of the analysis and the new understandings. Likewise, the participants in the research, whether they are clients or interviewees, can review the findings and add any additional insight and provide feedback to the researcher about his or her ability to understand the phenomenon being studied.

Finally, it is the researcher's job to present the findings to the community with enough detail and discussion for readers to understand the process involved as well as the meaning of the findings. Interestingly, in qualitative research, the burden of applicability of the findings to other phenomena is on the reader. If I read an ethnographic study of a group of adolescent girls with eating disorders in dance/movement therapy, it is up to me to determine whether the "truths" reported for this group have any impact for my own clinical work with adolescent girls.

PHENOMENOLOGICAL RESEARCH

What follows is a phenomenological study. First I will discuss phenomenology in general. Phenomenology is the study of human experience. As a phenomenologist, I do not evaluate experience as good or bad, or true or not true. I am most interested in simply understanding what people experience. As an example, imagine a veteran dance/movement therapist and a first-year graduate student in dance/movement therapy observing a session with a frail elder with severe cognitive and physical impairments. As one might guess, their observations would be quite different. The veteran dance/movement therapist might notice subtle movements in the client or small changes in the body posture while the student might be uncomfortable wondering why the therapist is working with a client who seems not to be even aware of her surroundings. Is one experience valid and the other not? Whose experience is correct? As a phenomenologist I am interested in both experiences. They are both "true" and valid. My goal in this example is to fully understand what the beginning student experiences when observing a session and also understand what the veteran dance/movement therapist experiences in a session. Further understanding both of these experiences is especially important if I am interested in having an impact on how dance/movement therapy is taught.

A Phenomenological Analysis of Dance/Movement Therapy with Frail Elders

I sought to understand or shed light on dance/movement therapy with frail elders. Given the elders' impairments, they were not able to self-report or provide information about what they experienced. Therefore I used the therapists as the research participants. In many instances, due to various impairments, clients may be unable to provide direct answers to questions about their experiences in therapy. Yet studying these experiences is critical, especially because therapists make decisions on the behalf of their clients. These decisions include determining which clients to treat, setting the goals and objectives, and deciding whether clients should be seen in individual or group therapy. Obviously, these decisions are made with as much information as possible.

Stance of the Researcher

During the course of this study I was working as a music therapist in the same facility and was familiar with the types of clients in the groups as well as the overall functioning of the facility. I brought to this study my own beliefs that the creative arts therapies can be very powerful in the treatment of frail elders. I also brought my values regarding the meaning of life for frail elders with multiple impairments. These values include honoring and respecting the client's humanity regardless of his or her level of functioning, and acknowledgment of an unknowable dimension to life, or an appreciation of the "implicate order" (Stige, 2002, p. 85).

Participants

Four therapists conducted six dance/movement therapy groups over a period of five months in a geriatric facility. The average age of group members was eighty-eight years and they ranged from mildly to severely physically and/or cognitively impaired. Groups in this study were composed of members with comparable abilities and/or deficits. The dance/movement therapists were all registered with the American Dance Therapy Association, had master's degrees, and had six to seventeen years of experience.

Method

The dance/movement therapists were asked to write narratives of each session, divided into three sections: a section relating goals, clinical observations, verbal and movement interventions, members' responses, et cetera; a section on personal reactions including feelings, observations, and intuitions; and a section containing general impressions. The narratives became the primary data for phenomenological analysis as applied by Giorgi (1984) and adapted by Forinash (1992). The analysis went as follows.

1. The researcher read each narrative to get an overall sense of the therapists' experiences.
2. Each narrative was reviewed multiple times with the researcher highlighting specific phrases or sentences that seemed significant. Attention was given to the phenomena as they appeared in the narrative rather than on assumptions of what the researcher expected to appear.
3. The highlighted phrases were transformed into themes or "meaning units" (Giorgi, 1984, p. 19).
4. Based on the meaning units, the researcher constructed a description of the therapists' experiences in dance/movement therapy with frail elders.
5. Meaning units and descriptions generated by the researcher were given to the therapists for clarification and feedback.
6. The researcher integrated the therapists' comments and feedback to create a comprehensive description of the therapists' experiences of dance/movement therapy with frail elders. This comprehensive description was submitted to the therapists. Their responses and additional comments were included in the conclusion section.

Results

During the data analysis of the therapists' narratives, the unifying theme that appeared was that of a continuum of "disconnectedness–connectedness." This specifically refers to how the therapists experienced the participation of their clients in the dance/movement therapy group. This continuum had both intrapersonal and interpersonal facets, reflecting the therapist's personal thoughts and experiences as well as experiences between members or between a member and the therapist. What follows are descriptions of experiences on this continuum, as well as excerpts from the therapists' narratives in italics, which provide a view of the raw data from which the results were derived. All participants have been given either a number or an initial as a means of providing anonymity.

Disconnectedness. At one end of the continuum was disconnectedness. On an intrapersonal level this was seen as a sense of disconnectedness from one's own feelings and memories. It almost seems that the clients feel they are not entitled or simply unwilling to experience their internal feelings and memories.

Therapist #1:
P said, "I don't really think this group is for us." When I pursued what she meant, she said she meant herself and the others in the group, that they were too old and "pirouettes" are silly things for them to be doing.

Therapist # 1:
We began with massaging hand lotion into our hands. After a moment, P said "Enough of this. This isn't important." I asked her what was important, but she was having difficulty with word finding. We took hands and I explained that we begin with massaging our hands as a reminder that we are taking care of our bodies.

On an interpersonal level it was seen as resistance to interacting with and connecting to other members, to the therapist, or to the dance/movement group.

Therapist # 2:
I felt hopeful about D joining; she had seemed so resistant. I worked hard *to get her in for the last two weeks. I also intercepted and encouraged L to attend and was frustrated not to get M to join. I am determined. I was struck by how isolated residents are and often occupied with ways to* not *connect. I felt hopeful (but worried) that we can perhaps address issues of isolation in the group. I wanted to increase horizontal movement and noticed resistance to this. R wouldn't reach to hold D's hand because she perceived D to be uninterested. They have real difficulty reaching out.*

Therapist #2
I tried to get the group to pass around leadership. N refused, F was confused, R did fine with it. The talk at the beginning really expressed the difficulty of this group forming a bond. One member said "I don't know anyone here." I replied "What about our group?" She replied "What group?"

Therapist #1
B said he would just watch. His eyes were glued to the paper he'd brought. When I asked questions, he was amicable and answered. He said yes, he stretched by bending over . . . but no he didn't want to do it now.

Connectedness. At the other end of the continuum was connectedness. On an intrapersonal level this was evidenced when the group member connected to a memory imbued with emotion through movement experiences, or gained some level of insight and personal awareness that impacted on his/her present life.

Therapist #1:
We then began to move hands and I asked what activities they did with their hands. R said reaching for the gold ring on the carousel. This led to a discussion where each remembered carousel riding. P laughed as she said she'd fallen off trying a couple of times. M said she hadn't tried because she didn't want to lose her seat. R said she had caught it a couple of times, winning a free ride and that she had been showing off, trying to be better than the others.

Therapist #2:
We did a punching movement which I got from seeing N's fist as we stretched arms upward. This led to a discussion of R feeling powerless to punch because her wrists are so thin, but acknowledging her strength when she feels mad. . . . R said "If you are mad let it be known!"

Therapist #1:
I asked B to lead a movement or stretch that feels good. B said "A movement that I used to do that gave me the greatest feeling of zest in my life was simonizing my car. It's really silly. . . ." I asked B to show us just how he did it. He demonstrated that he took stuff out of the jar and put it on the car and then rubbed it in. . . . Everyone did the movement. . . . I said that while I didn't expect he was going to re-experience the zest he'd felt at 25 now at 90 years of age but that by doing that movement he would feel more zest than he'd felt one hour before.

Therapist #3:
They chose soft music today . . . the music was so moving to S that she spent some time crying and remembering old times. She wouldn't share her memories but said they were personal. Her body and whole affect indulged in the memory and she moved beautifully, expanding her body in the space above her, beside her and in front of her.

The following excerpt is from a group with a greater number of physical and cognitive impairments that made it more challenging to engage verbally.

Therapist #4:
It was nice at the end, we did breathing exercises and a balloon image was created. It seemed that both E and M had a profound sense of release as we let our imaginary balloons blow up and then float off. They both seemed to lift and release their chest and neck area. M actually commented that it "felt good." E kept her arms in a sustained hold out to the side as she closed her eyes and took a few more deep breaths.

The following excerpt examines the change in internal experiences that occurred in this group.

Therapist #3:

I asked them to name their feeling and then, using movement and gestures, show the group how they were feeling. E "lousy" her head and arms dropped. B "sleepy and deject-ed," she folded her body over and sighed. F "good," she bounced her shoulders and sat up. J "sleepy," he leaned his head on his hand. S "tired," she leaned way over and put her hands against her head and rocked from side to side.

Later in the same session:

We did another check in at the end. I asked them to show us in their bodies. B sat up tall and lifted her chin. E raised her arms up. F did the same and shook her shoulders. J used his arms as though he were climbing a rope. S sat up tall, swayed and looked side to side. J stated "I feel alive now."

On an interpersonal level, a connection was made in or through move-ment between members or between a member and the therapist. For clients with less impairment, the movement engendered respect, recognition, and appreciation for each other. Even members with severe impairments had moments of awareness and recognition of others.

Therapist #2:
The slow, easy rhythm of the music was a good tempo to sway and push hands in the cen-ter, making circles. We mostly just held hands and swayed. We talked a lot about suffer-ing—dealing with certain levels of acceptance of it. There was much more support of each other. That was wonderful! Moods really brightened, I think, because of the connection.

Therapist #1:
I asked them if they would like to continue with the balloon or use scarves. R said scarves. The music ended with M, who had been singing along with the music. She began to hum. We all hummed together and M made up words as though to a lullaby. S and P laughed and joined in. We moved the scarves to the music and then again explored them as veils.

For more severely impaired clients, there were moments of simple recog-nition of others as members toss a balloon in rhythm for several minutes.

Therapist #4:
I put on music and began tossing the balloon. There was an immediate sense of com-munity and clients were using arms and feet to toss the balloon . . . we were able to main-tain a unified rhythm for four clients for a few minutes. . . . I noticed that postures did shift to an increase in vertical.

Given the level of disability of many of the members in this group, the dance/movement therapist was clearly moved by the interpersonal connec-tion that occurs through the movement.

Therapist #3:
For a moment three members were moving cohesively, four including me, and I even asked these three clients to initiate a movement and said we would follow. It worked. I don't remember this ever happening in this group before where one person led and oth-ers followed—and I mean others with an s! It was wonderful!

Conclusions

The results discussed above were submitted to the dance/movement therapists for their comments and responses. They agreed that the results accurately reflected their experiences. They commented that it was interesting to read one another's experiences and it was affirming to see the similarities.

Therapist #1 pointed out that P in her groups was noted by nursing staff to have no short-term memory, yet participated quite appropriately in the group. Staff often had to help P with her meals because she could not remember the function of her fork, knife, or plate.

Yet P remembered the group members and myself each week and asked about those not present. She even remembered that I was going to Europe after the end of the group and reminded me and the group about that. Her short-term memory in fact, seemed quite good when it was about people in this small, consistent group.

Therapist #4 responded to the theme of connectedness.

It is interesting—the process you used—how you came up with connectedness. It makes sense and is truly a basic element in our work. It also got me thinking of other areas and other kinds of connections. . . . I thought specifically of the kind of connections made with and throughout the body—integration of and use of the full body and genuine movements. I like the internal/external connectedness. I am actually very excited to see our work coming together so nicely and making sense.

Therapist #1 also resonated with the concept of connectedness.

This is clear and essential. I love that connectedness came out as a key concept. This research provides a very nurturing feel to our work. I have two more thoughts. 1) I am aware all the more of how we (our culture) and even I sometimes ignore or devalue the process of relationship which is manifested in the body movement often in the spaces between the words. How we value labeling and talking about things more than simply being. 2) I am reminded of a lesson which I have to keep relearning and which I think dance/movement therapy process directly teaches and confronts—that there is no place like the present. If you get stuck in a place and breathe into it and move in it authentically you will move to the next natural place.

This study has brought to light the theme of the continuum of disconnectedness-connectedness in the work of these dance/movement therapists with frail elders. This continuum has both intrapersonal and interpersonal aspects. Intrapersonally, disconnectedness can be demonstrated by resistances to one's own internal experiences, feelings, and memories. Interpersonally, disconnectedness can be demonstrated by a resistance to acknowledge or connect with other members or the therapist.

Intrapersonally, connectedness can be seen as an experience of one's personal past and can include happy memories and associations as well as painful associations. Interpersonally, connectedness allows members to engage and interact with each other and can occur regardless of the level of functioning of the clients. This interpersonal connectedness allows members to have a thorough, integrated sense of themselves, and creates the potential for fuller relationships with others.

Therapist #1 demonstrates in her narrative the power of the movement to create a poignant sense of internal connectedness.

We had been moving our shoulders. I talked about the importance of moving shoulders back to counteract the effects of aging on the spine. I talked about the wings (scapulas). M said "We'll need these later so that we can fly." I repeated it with a questioning intonation. M replied "When we fly to heaven."

DISCUSSION

What follows is a brief discussion of the theoretical points raised early in this chapter regarding positions of ontology, epistemology, and methodology; issues of trustworthiness; guidelines for interviewing and observing; and procedures of data and how those points were addressed in the phenomenological research presented.

This phenomenological research clearly falls into the constructivist *ontology*. There is no search for absolute or relative truth here, as well as no discussion of social context and values. The researcher sought to understand the experience of dance/movement therapy with frail elders. *Epistemologically*, the researcher's questions were not about effectiveness but about how the therapists experienced working with the frail elders and what meaning they made of this work, and the therapists' narratives constituted knowledge to inform the questions. *Methodologically* the researcher chose phenomenology, not to evaluate the therapists' effectiveness, but rather to understand and shed light on their experience.

Issues of *trustworthiness* were addressed in several ways. Falling under the area of Bruscia's (1998) *personal integrity*, the researcher shared her biases at the beginning of the study so the reader could understand her basic values and beliefs. Regarding the area of *interpersonal integrity*, the researcher appears to have had a positive working relationship with the therapists evidenced by the depth of their personal thoughts and comments in the process notes. In the area of *methodological integrity* the researcher submitted the data analysis to the therapists for their responses and suggestions. *Aesthetic integrity* is best evaluated by those reading this chapter.

Interviewing and *observing* were not used in this example as the researcher used the session narratives written by the therapists as the data. The structure of the narrative was meant to be inclusive of many of the questions covered earlier in this chapter and include goals, observations (*descriptive questions*), interventions (*example questions*), members' responses' (*clarification questions*), personal reactions, feelings, and intuitions (*paradigmatic questions*), and general impressions (*closing questions*).

Data analysis followed a general form of *deconstruction* (analysis of each narrative multiple times); *generation of meaning units or themes* (continuum of connectedness with examples from the narratives); and *reconstruction* (thorough description of the continuum of disconnectedness–connectedness with both intrapersonal and interpersonal aspects).

Readers are encouraged to read research with an awareness of the general areas presented above. While not all researchers articulate their ontological position, they likely will include how they dealt with issues of trustworthiness, what their interview questions were, and how they analyzed their data.

FINAL THOUGHTS

Qualitative research is providing and will continue to provide a unique and meaningful way in which to further understand clients' experiences, clinical practice, and the field of dance/movement therapy and the other creative arts therapies. Clearly, these fields will continue to develop and use research methods that allow creative arts therapists to understand, as fully as possible, the meaning of the work that they are committed to do.

REFERENCES

Aigen, K. (1991). *The roots of music therapy: Towards an indigenous research paradigm.* (Doctoral Dissertation, New York University.) UMI order # 9134717.

Aigen, K. (1993). The music therapist as qualitative researcher. *Music Therapy, 12(1)* 16–39.

Aigen, K. (1996). *Being in music. Foundations of Nordoff-Robbins music therapy.* St. Louis, MO: MMB Music.

Aigen, K. (1997). *Here we are in music: One year with an adolescent creative music therapy group.* St. Louis, MO: MMB Music.

Aigen, K. (1998). *Paths of development in Nordoff-Robbins music therapy.* Gilsum, NH: Barcelona Publishers.

American Psychological Association. (2001). *Publication manual of the American Psychological Association* (5th ed). Washington, DC: Author.

Amir, D. (1996). Experiencing music therapy: Meaningful moments in the music therapy process. In M. Langenberg, K. Aigen, & J. Frommer (Eds.), *Qualitative music therapy research: Beginning dialogues.* Gilsum, NH: Barcelona Publishers.

Bartenieff, I., Davis, M., & Paulay, F. (1970). *Four adaptations of effort theory in research and teaching.* New York: Dance Notation Bureau.

Blumenefeld-Jones, D. S. (1995). Dance as a mode of research representation. *Qualitative Inquiry, 1*(4), 391–401.

Bruscia, K. E. (1995). Modes of consciousness in Guided Imagery and Music (GIM): A therapist's experience of the guiding process. In C. B. Kenny (Ed.), *Listening, playing creating: Essays on the power of sound.* Albany, NY: State University of New York Press.

Bruscia, K. E. (1998). Standards of integrity for qualitative music therapy research. *Journal of Music Therapy, 35*(3), 176–200.

Creswell, J. W. (1998). *Qualitative inquiry and research design: Choosing among five traditions.* Thousand Oaks, CA: Sage.

Edwards, J. (1999). Considering the paradigmatic frame: Social science research approaches relevant to research in music therapy. *The Arts in Psychotherapy, 26*(2), 73–80.

Forinash, M. (1992). A phenomenological analysis of Nordoff-Robbins approach to music therapy: The lived experience of clinical improvisation. *Music Therapy, 11*(1), 120–141.

Forinash, M. (1993). An exploration into qualitative research in music therapy. *The Arts in Psychotherapy, 20*(1), 69–73.

Forinash, M., & Lee, C. (1998). Guest editorial. *Journal of Music Therapy, 35*(3), 142–149.

Giorgi, A. (1984). A phenomenological psychological analysis of the artistic process. In J.G. Gilbert (Ed.), *Qualitative evaluation in the arts, II.* New York: New York University School of Education, Health, Nursing and Arts Professions.

Guba, E. G. (1990). The alternative paradigm dialog. In E.G. Guba (Ed.), *The paradigm dialog.* Thousand Oaks, CA: Sage.

Guba, E. G., & Lincoln, Y. (1994). Competing paradigms in qualitative research. In N. K. Denzin and Y. S. Lincoln (Eds.), *Handbook of qualitative research.* Thousand Oaks, CA: Sage.

Hervey, L.W. (2000). *Artistic inquiry in dance/movement therapy: Creative alternatives for research.* Springfield, IL: Charles C Thomas.

Higgens, L. (2000). On the value of conducting dance/movement therapy research. *The Arts in Psychotherapy, 27*(1), 191–196.

Janesick, V. J. (1998). *"Stretching" exercises for qualitative researchers.* Thousand Oaks, CA: Sage.

Laban, R. (1960). *The mastery of movement.* London: MacDonald & Evans.

Laban, R., & Lawrence, F.C. (1947). *Effort.* New York: Dance Horizons.

Lewis, P., & Loman, S. (1990). *The Kestenberg movement profile: Its past, present applications and future directions.* Keene, NH: Antioch New England Graduate School.

Lincoln, Y., & Guba, E. (1985). *Naturalistic inquiry.* Thousand Oaks, CA: Sage.

McNiff, S. (1998). *Art-based research.* London: Jessica Kingsley.

Moustakes, C. (1961). *Loneliness.* Englewood Cliffs, NJ: Prentice-Hall.

Moustakes, C. (1972). *Loneliness and love.* Englewood Cliffs, NJ: Prentice-Hall.

Moustakes, C. (1975). *The touch of loneliness.* Englewood Cliffs, NJ: Prentice-Hall.

Moustakes, C. (1990). *Heuristic research: Design, methodology and application.* Thousand Oaks, CA: Sage.

Reynolds, F. (2000). Managing depression through needlecraft creative activities: A qualitative study. *The Arts in Psychotherapy, 27*(1), 107–114.

Sandel, S. L., Chaiklin, S., & Lohn, A. (1993). *Foundations of dance/movement therapy: The life and work of Marian Chace.* Columbia, MD: The Marian Chace Memorial Fund.

Spaniol, S. (1998). Towards an ethnographic approach to art therapy research: People with psychiatric disability as collaborators. *Art Therapy: Journal of the American Art Therapy Association, 15*(1), 29–37.

Stige, B. (2002). Do we need general criteria for the evaluation of qualitative research? *Nordic Journal of Music Therapy, 11*(1), 65–71.

Wheeler, B. (Ed.), (1995). *Music therapy research: Quantitative and qualitative perspectives.* Gilsum, NH: Barcelona Publishers.

Chapter 9

APPLYING ANTHROPOLOGICAL METHODS IN DANCE/MOVEMENT THERAPY RESEARCH

JUDITH LYNNE HANNA

Why apply anthropological methods in dance/movement therapy research? I will begin to address this issue by presenting a current example of the need for healing in the increasingly multicultural United States facing posttraumatic stress anxiety and disorder. This example of the need for posttraumatic stress therapy is but one example within the broad spectrum of uses of dance/movement therapy. Then, given the essential role of nonverbal communication in the dance/movement therapy process, I address how the anthropological approach can help to discover the ways in which different groups communicate nonverbally on the basis of their cultural beliefs and how this can affect the cause and cure of mental and emotional problems. I will describe methods anthropologists use to discover differences, similarities, and dance/movement-specific analytic frameworks and categories that can usefully be applied in dance/movement therapy research.

AN ILLUSTRATIVE NEED

September 11, 2001: horrific unprecedented terrorism. Nearly 3,000 people gruesomely killed at the World Trade Center in New York City as two hijacked American planes crashed into the majestic twin towers. People from eighty countries lost their lives. Terrorists also flew an American plane to Pennsylvania where passengers forced the plane to crash into a field to avoid hitting an unknown target. All on board died. Terrorists crashed a fourth plane into the Pentagon in Washington, D.C., demolishing one of its walls into a pile of rubbish. Americans find it hard to fathom their vulnerability in the most powerful nation in the world.

The sheer scale of 9-11 managed to dwarf mental health professional resources (Goode & Eakin, 2002). Trauma experts were in demand. Mental health practitioners were needed in family assistance centers, offices, schools, psychiatric hospitals, clinics, and communities. The emotional force was so strong that even people accustomed to coping on their own sought help.

144

In anxious times, people experience posttraumatic stress syndrome, emotional distress, and other emotional disorders that interfere with functioning. Ripples of tragedy and uncertainty, shock and sadness, fear and helplessness are felt. Reported symptoms of post-traumatic stress disorder can include reliving the trauma, sleepless nights, nightmares, irritability, overindulgence in work, drugs, or food, distancing from intimates, nonspecific ailments, depression, acting out, startle responses, withdrawal, fearfulness, anxiety, outbreaks of rage, trembling, tics, aversion to body parts or bodily functions, dissociation, alteration of identity, and repetitive behavior.

Traumas often lead to refugee, runaway, or other kinds of homeless status. Violence inflicted by human beings can exact a greater psychic toll than the impersonal cruelty of nature (Gray, 2001). People with prior psychiatric conditions who had been improving frequently have setbacks as a result of violence. The impact of distress is often exacerbated by other stresses, such as loss of jobs and displacement from homes.

HEALING

Among its many uses, dance/movement therapy aims to help people overcome trauma, often by bringing the elements of the experience to the fore nonverbally in order to work through them. This means to engage in a process in which they face the same trauma under a therapist's guidance until they are able to overcome the stress. A retelling, giving testimony, can help to make sense of the incomprehensible and transform the surreal into something real. Under the protective cloak of therapy, clients who suffer bewilderment, dislocation, and revisited negative emotions from traumatic stress can access resources that help them to transform these feelings. Aggressively motivated pain inflicted on the body usually requires a restoration of the sense of accepting the "dirtied" body, integration of the separated body and soul, and rebuilding social relationships (see Bernstein, 1995; Chang & Leventhal, 1995; Hanna, 1995; Liebmann, 1996; Frank, 1997; Graessner, Gurris, & Pross, 2001; Gray, 2001; Landy, 2002).

Nonverbal communication, the bodily sending and receiving of messages, is integral to the dance/movement healing process and makes it unique among Western forms of therapy. Over the years, America has welcomed refugees from many troubled places in the world—Europe, Latin America, Vietnam, Cambodia, Somalia, Ethiopia, El Salvador, Nepal, and Pakistan, to name but a few. There is internal diversity within national groups based, for example, on religion, language, ethnicity, economics, gender, age, social status, and immigration period (see Foner, 2001; Zephir, 2001). There are involuntary minorities, groups that did not choose to become part of the U.S. but were forced against their will. These minorities include American

Indians, Alaskan natives, early Mexican Americans in the Southwest, native Hawaiians, Puerto Ricans, and black Americans brought to the United States as slaves. The ways they have interpreted and responded to their situation of mistreatment by white Americans affect their attitude to white institutions/practices. Their individual and community's experiences with segregation, racism, job and other economic discrimination have led to distrust of white institutions/practices and exhibition of defensive, oppositional behavior. Speaking standard English, for example, is seen as giving in to the white oppressor and abandoning one's group identity. Ogbu and Simons (1998) point out: "Some beliefs and behaviors apply to enough members of a minority group or a type of minority group to form a visible pattern," (p. 168). But, "not all members of a minority group believe the same thing or behave the same way" (p. 168). And change occurs.

Does the nonverbal communication of these groups vary distinctively in some ways? Given that verbal languages and cultures differ, it seems probable that people would differentially experience and cope with trauma and express emotions. Each emotion has its own characteristics, and there are different ways of working with each. Specific movement patterns that correlate with particular core emotional syndromes may vary culturally.

Culture, a social heritage of values, beliefs, and ways of doing things that people learn from each other and through which they adapt and adjust to the external world and to each other, has two aspects. One is the observed manifestations including actions, gestures, and pictures. The other is the mental world of meanings and understandings. Thomas (2001), for example, showed differences in conceptions of reality, living things, knowing, cause, competence, innate characteristics, attributes of self, esteemed traits, consequences of behavior, values, and prohibitions; others also showed different conceptions of health, illness, and healing (Acosta, Yamamoto, & Evans, 1982; Atkinson, Martin, & Sue, 1989; Boddy, 1988; Friedson, 1996; Guindy & Schmais, 1994; Hanna, 1995; Helman, 2000; Ho, 1987; Janzen, 2002; Kleinman, 1980, 1995; Madsen, 1973; McElroy & Townsend, 1989; Nichter & Lock, 2002).

However, culture does not maintain a coherent static and unchanging set of values. Culture is porous to outside influences and pressures. It often incorporates competing repertoires of meaning and action.

Not only is the United States multicultural, but dance/movement therapy has spread to thirty-one countries throughout the world (Dosamantes-Beaudry, 1999). So anthropological research may serve to moderate the misinterpretation of behavior of people from different cultures and groups "read" from traditional dance/movement therapy perspectives that first developed in the 1940s. Many practitioners may have assumed that Western cultural underpinnings and manifestations of emotion were universal. Yet anthropological research has challenged the assumption of universality (Hanna, 1983, 1990, 1995, 2002a). So, it is important to question Euro-

American patterns rather than project them onto other groups; to present them as hypotheses and not a priori assumptions.

Of key importance to dance/movement therapists is that effective communication depends on shared meanings, including expectations about what a form of communication should encompass. Dance/movement therapists, therefore, seek to understand the meaning of their clients' movements. But what if the symbolism is culturally specific? Sometimes clients identify with the bad guy to make them feel powerful and in control. Again, what if the identification symbolism is culturally specific? People who have not been given choices in life may find it overwhelming, intimidating, and stressful to make choices about how they want to express and validate themselves in therapy.

If clients encounter their own culturally relevant nonverbal communication in a therapeutic setting, they are more likely to trust therapy and consider it legitimate. Awareness of cultural rules for verbal and nonverbal social engagement shows respect for the client's traditional life style. Ignorance subverts healing efforts. Scaffolding therapy on cultural norms is more likely to lead to success and avoidance of new stress.

KEY QUESTIONS

Anthropological research methods can be used to discover, for example, to what extent the theories and methods accepted in dance/movement therapy to deal with stress are applicable to different cultures. People have multiple identities, so which set of beliefs and practices do they rely on during difficult times? What stimuli do different groups consider traumatic? How are they expected to cope in response to trauma? Does religion help? How? How do people display and identify different emotions? Under what circumstances? With what result?

What do different peoples believe cause illness, its manifestation and cure? What are their healing practices? How are these initiated? What are the career motivations and restraints to becoming a healer who uses dance/movement therapeutically? Many people find succor in religion and dance/movement is part of religious practice in many parts of the world.

Culturally sensitive dance/movement therapy would also ask: How do various groups view the body, dance/movement, and dance with members of the opposite sex or different status? Do people touch? Who, when, where, how, how strongly, and for how long? Is touching ritual, affect, play, or control? What are the preferred spatial relationships between people?

What variables in dance/movement preserve, promote, or change ideas or identities? What is the impact on others than the client in a dance/movement therapy situation? What wisdom and practices do other people have that dance/movement therapists can benefit from?

Among many people, altered body and mind states are not subsumed under a biologically derived vocabulary and world-view. Sickness for them is the result of specific events and changes. Health and illness involve not only body functions but also interpersonal relationships, cultural values, emotions, religious, political, economic, and environmental factors that impinge on an individual and groups. For example, says Rubenstein (2002):

> Just as we believe in microbes, which can only be seen by people trained to use the proper equipment, Shuar [in Ecuador] believe in things they call *tsentsak* (which they translate as 'darts') that only shamans can see. We believe that microbes can be manipulated to harm others, through biological warfare— but we also believe that they act on their own, and that illness usually occurs independent of any human agency. Shuar, however, believe that *tsentsak* act only through human agency, and that all such illness is actually the result of an intentional act of violence. People will thus explain illness in terms of pre-existing tensions or conflicts between the victim and others, and illness could provoke some act of vengeance. Shuar thus link physical disease to social unease (p. 1).

Medical anthropology recognizes that culture plays a role in shaping people's attitudes toward health. Care behaviors that appear inexplicable or inappropriate to Western eyes may stem from beliefs that clients hold to be reasonable and well founded.

Clearly, information from anthropological approaches to uncovering meaning in movement, dance, health, and healing can inform clinical practice with heterogeneous populations. Anthropology respects the aesthetic and humanistic nature of dance/movement therapy and can often identify what kinds of questions can be quantitatively researched. Since the 1920s, numerous anthropologists have contributed a substantial literature on dance and also on health and healing.

ANTHROPOLOGY

The questions concerning multicultural nonverbal communication and trauma can be investigated anthropologically to gain a nuanced understanding of people's beliefs and practices that impact on their inner lives and movement expression. Anthropologists try to understand how and why cultures are similar and different. Seeking to understand a group's dance/movement, anthropologists view it within a holistic perspective that fits it and its context (ecology) together within a whole. Dance/movement is produced by a complex interaction of artistic and social processes. Not an isolated act, dance/movement is intertwined with the culture of a people living together with a history in a geographical space.

Researchers have demonstrated that we must turn to society and not just to the dancer's experience to understand the meaning of dance. It reflects social forces and relates to a larger domain of movement. At the same time, however, dance may be more than epiphenomenal and serve as a vehicle through which individuals influence social forces and behavior. That is, dance may reflect what is and also *influence what might be* (Hanna, 1987, 1988a, 1988b).

Anthropologists look at the dance itself, its movement and meaning, as well as its participants, setting, and history. Anthropologists ascertain dancers' intentions, the viewers' and others' perceptions, and what the participants in a dance event both say and do. Anthropologists also examine how the actions fit into the broader context of society, culture, and history.

Theory guides informed exploration. The Processual Model of Dance, Figure 9-1 (Hanna, 1987), illustrates the complexity and directs attention to phenomena to explore. For a dance performance there is a catalyst (A) determining who dances, why, where, and how vis-à-vis cultural values, society, polity, economy, and religion. For example, a village market, family birth or death, or festival makes participation in an Ubakala (Igbo group in Nigeria) dance virtually obligatory for performers and spectators. Individual or group initiative to conserve social patterns, introduce change, or cope with the behavioral exaggeration of a contradictory principle in the Ubakala ethos stimulates yet another performance. Selective perception (B) is the extraction of information from sensory stimulation on the basis of memory and cognitive structures, emotion, hereditary capabilities, learned communication skill, and sociocultural experience. Ubakala motivations, incentives, and desired reward of participating in a dance include the fear of being shamed for not meeting expectations, pleasure, social approval, prestige and/or money received for a praiseworthy performance, and the need to keep informed of current events conveyed through the performance. The dancer, an incumbent of a social role, selectively perceives the situation and makes movement choices with some intention (B) to inform, evaluate, prescribe, and/or affect; or without specific intention, but with the possibility that information transfer may occur. Intent becomes transformed through the communication medium (C) of the dance. Performers encode messages through devices which operate in one or more spheres with rules governing the combination of these elements through the dance channel (see discussion below of probing for meaning in movement). There may be adjunct channels such as music, song, and costume. The arrows in the model suggest feedback possibilities such as introducing information about a performance in the performance, to reinforce or change it. Natural events such as rain or a fight may interfere with the dance. There is a catalyst for the audience to attend a dance. The audience interprets the message (D) with selective perception. The dance may have implications for the dancer, observers, and what catalyzed the dance in the first place.

Viewing dance as a key medium of communication, a way people represent themselves to themselves and to each other, dance may be a sign of itself, a sign with referents beyond itself, and an instrument, such as a means

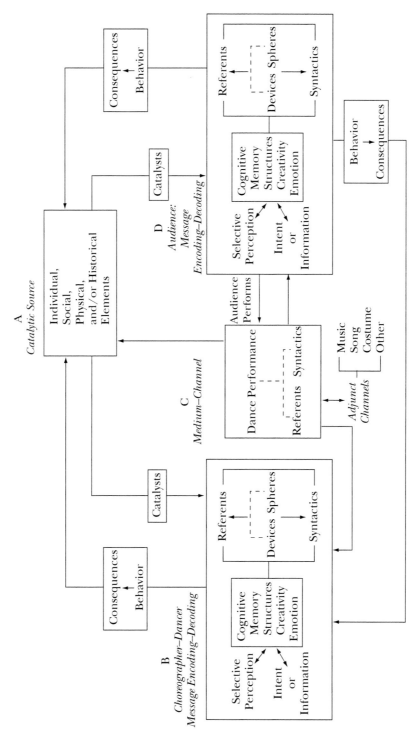

Figure 9-1   Processual Model of Dance: Phenomena to Explore in the Process and Performance of Dance

to promote healing (Hanna, 1987, 2001; Sebeok, 2001). Language-like, dance usually assembles its linguistic-like elements in a manner that more often resembles poetry, with its suggestive imagery, rhythm, ambiguity, multiple meanings, and latitude in form. Because a symbol condenses a number of affectively linked associations, it has an affective charge. Perhaps this is why dance has long held pride of place in religion, ethnic identity, gender, and social stratification.

The optical array of danced signs may lead to reinforcing ongoing patterns of social behavior or acquiring new responses. Alternatively, the danced signs may lead to weakening or strengthening inhibitions over fully elaborated patterns in a person's repertoire. In addition, the danced signs may lead to facilitating performance of previously learned behavior that was encumbered by restraints.

Anthropologists usually focus on a group with a shared culture, their own or another's. Learning about a culture, and being aware that intra-cultural differences exist (for example by, sex, gender, age, social class, ethnicity, race, occupational group, knowledge, and personality), anthropologists seek to discover, record, analyze, and then "translate" the perspectives of different members of a group and convey this knowledge. Process oriented, anthropologists engage in dialogic editing with the culture they study. That is, they maintain a healthy skepticism about knowledge claims and rule out alternative explanations. Anthropologists elicit feedback to verify their interpretations from the client group and their professional peers, and modify their interpretations as necessary.

Anthropologists draw upon whatever methods they deem most useful to explore theoretically based questions. This means they use quantitative or qualitative methods, or a combination of both (Bernard, 2000, 2001; Hanna, 1983; Altamira Press and Sage Publications have many relevant methods books). Researchers indicate what historical documents they investigated and state their sources of contemporary information: how many people they observed and interviewed and how representative these people are of a group. Anthropology recognizes that fieldworkers are not neutral, invisible conduits mechanically recording "facts" and "truths" with objective, ideological neutralism. So researchers try to identify their biases and personal decisions in unexpected and conflictual situations. Reflexivity to expose personal motives, emotions, and beliefs creates the context for the pursuit of "truths" and an account that allows the reader to understand the researcher's position in it. Of course, all research methods have limitations, and I will point out some of these.

Ethnographic Method: Participant-Observation

The serious noncorrespondence between laboratory and naturalistic measures of the "same" behavior leads anthropologists to engage in ethnography, a form of qualitative research methodology that seeks to understand the perspectives and practices of groups of people by close and direct contact. Ethnography is carried out in naturalistic settings where observation and interviewing take place and events occur.

Participant-observation developed as a reaction to speculative history, armchair guessing. Ethnographers place themselves among the people they are trying to understand, asking questions and observing in much the same way as a child learns its culture. Detailed field notes, photographs, audiotaped interviews, and filmed or videotaped movement comprise key data.

The human instrument is a research tool, interacting with subjects, as therapists interact with clients. However, entering a group's life can never fully give the outsider an understanding of their experiences. Inevitably, the participant-observer has an effect on the people and situations observed as well as being affected by them.

Although subjectivity is inherent in ethnography, the researcher strives to set aside preconceptions and to be systematic. Self-knowledge accrues during research. However, the goal is to understand the perspective of the other, not the researcher's own self. In a creative process, anthropologists seek facts and truth from the participant's and the participant's associates' perspectives. The process of making sense and discovering meaning from interviews and observations is a search for patterns and relationships in order to describe complex phenomena, generate theoretical models, and reframe questions. Ethnographers try to clarify conditions and contexts that may shape causal connections in social and behavioral queries.

Dance/movement therapists would most likely select groups to study from which they have clients, groups not studied, or groups not served or underserved. Because anthropological methods can be used to understand cultures, another tack might be to consider the dance/movement therapy profession as a culture and study it; or to define a diagnostic group as a culture and attempt to study how dance/movement therapy is viewed in this culture. Yet another topic might be comparing dance/movement therapy cultures as they exist internationally. Practitioners are members of indigenous cultures in their homelands who may adapt dance/movement therapy practice to their culture. (See below on intra-cultural variation; also, Jacobs-Huey, 2002, on how education may make an insider an outsider.)

Entering a group's community can be facilitated by a member of the group introducing the ethnographer, or knowing people who know people inside the group. Self-introduction and explanation of one's purpose is another way to gain access. There are, of course, issues concerning protecting informants and in some cultures one must gain permission from elders or men to talk to young people and women.

Time and event sampling can be used to learn about each of several different groups' patterns of dance/movement, emotional expression, and views about healing. Patterns can be sought in television and movies about the groups, in addition to the clients' family at home and in the neighborhood, church, school, park, and market.

Getting several accounts or descriptions of the same event or person is one of the defining features of field work. Multiple accounts allow a triangulation of the truth. Sometimes different reports appear as irreducibly different visions of a reality. Then anthropologists analyze the relation between what people do and what they say and the context of history and environment.

Historical Grounding

Following the anthropological approach requires first examining literature, archival material, and artifacts related to the group they plan to study. Ethnographers try to learn as much as possible prior to interaction with members of a group in order to be aware of customs and sensitivities. Moreover, because a culture's dance/movement is transmitted from one generation to the next, history provides a base line to observe change. The Human Relations Area Files provide a database of ethnographic material. Other scholars may have useful unpublished materials. Talking with former dance/movement therapy clients about their experiences can provide another source of historical grounding.

Client Group Views

Client views are important to discover in and of themselves, as well as to modify the analyst's conceptual and comparative categories. Ways of questioning can determine answers. Field interview procedures may use non-translational linguistics (tell me about), interactive elicitation (what is it, what is it called) or word-to-text elicitation of the name of a phenomenon and asking a person to discuss it.

Yet reliance upon an informant's verbal exegesis alone for description and analysis may preclude understanding some people's dance/movement. The language of dance is nonverbal and not always easily translatable into words. Many features of dance lie beyond the conscious awareness of dancers and viewers. In numerous cultures, dancers do not know or have names for specific dance steps. Just as grammarians and linguists are knowledgeable about vocabulary and syntax, and psychologists understand emotions and how they are expressed, so movement analysts are familiar with comparable elements in dance.

However, if a culture does not analyze the dance it performs, a researcher must then rely upon the disciplinary heritage in relevant scholarly fields (Hanna, 1989a, 1989b). This is the case even though a scholarly approach may be Western and have an ethnocentric bias. Of course, researchers should elicit feedback on their analyses from representatives of the groups whose dances they study and modify their analyses as appropriate. Note that when a group does not have verbalized aesthetic views about its dance culture, the researcher's intervention in trying to elicit verbalization rather than observe activity may trigger a new concept that is the researcher's artifact.

Krebs (1975), in a valuable approach followed by other anthropologists, used film playback of Thai dance for Thai informants to elicit meaning from their perspectives. Film provides a specific focus to reinforce the verbal and to help a researcher uncover areas she or he is not aware of. Film can be run at normal speed, frozen at any particular point, projected in slow motion or repeated over and over again. The native informant may correct the filmmaker-researcher: "You missed the important part, your camera should have been pointing over here to the right." Krebs filmed a Khon masked dance-drama performance and interviewed Thais, both experts and laymen. Film/videotape elicitation is based on theories of ethnoscience concerning how members of a culture conceptualize and structure the world they live in. Rather than ask "what story is this?" she would ask "what is happening?" Rather than ask "what is the name of this dance?" (which assumes the existence of "dance"), she asked "what is this called?" giving the informant the opportunity to interpret "this."

Even when an informant comments on dance/movement, it may be difficult to know what actually is being said. Words often have multiple meanings; things taken for granted may not be articulated; lies, rationalizations, jokes, and metaphors are possibilities. Like poetry, dance is often layered with many meanings, and like a Rorschach inkblot test, each person interprets dance on the basis of individual experience, situation, and culturally-influenced perception.

Body Knowledge

Anthropologists have performed the dances of an indigenous person to elicit the group's aesthetics. But this is problematic, because what suffices for an outsider may be an inadequate performance for an insider. And criteria for insiders may differ according to age, gender, or other category.

Contemporary dance research recognizes sensuous epistemologies, a corporeal mode of knowing, and mind/body integration of cognition, feeling, and emotion that constitute realities for both performers and perceivers. Some researchers reflexively use their own bodily movement experience, looking at the self inside out with internal awareness and viewing the body from a first person perception. However, using this experiential bodily practice to privilege subjective experience as if it were that of another person's dance to describe the way sensation is organized and felt by that person, especially of a different culture or group within one's own culture, is speculative, narcissistic, and ethnocentric. In fact, it silences the other (Salzman, 2002). Self-reporting on the part of the researcher may be contaminated with wish fulfillment. Moreover, not all of one's critical personal life is available to consciousness. Everyone carries a distinct repertoire of psychobiological responses, cultural understandings, and beliefs.

Recording Physical Movement

Dance or movement research requires competence in movement analysis. One can learn the concepts of a notation system without using the notation itself. Verbalizing movement analysis allows the broader dissemination of dance research.

Anthropologists observe and record dance to provide semantic data that can be used by itself or in conjunction with dance participants' (producers', performers', and spectators') views. A problem is that seeing is creating meaning. Even highly trained movement analysts may vary in their perceptions, interpretations, and notations of a dance. Accurate and speedy notation of dance in its field context is difficult. The reason is that some dances may be performed only once during a researcher's visit, and some dancers may be unable or unwilling to replicate a performance. Rather than being raw data, notation is a translation. Thus to make the dance more objectively accessible, researchers often preserve dance behavior on film and video. Use of film and video makes actions more objectively accessible and permits valid and reliable analysis and reanalysis of units of movement in slow motion, in much the same way a sociolinguist or a musicologist might use a tape recording to prepare a transcript (see Hanna, 1989a). Grid-marked lenses allow detailed movement analysis as in Olympics training research. Of course, film is two-dimensional, not palpably three-dimensional, and there is selectivity in what is filmed and how. Consequently, an ideal situation would involve several cameras to obtain different perspectives and samples of time and place.

"How will a simple notation which is sophisticated in the interpretation of form account for the empirical content of . . . a dance?" asks Layiwola (1999, p. 7). He faults Western notation for being unable to deal with empathy and story line. I faced such a question when I began my first fieldwork in 1962 among the Ubakala Igbo of Nigeria.

PROBING FOR MEANING IN MOVEMENT

Anthropological field work among the Ubakala Igbo of Nigeria, in 1962, and then further analyses of their dances between 1973 and 1976, made me realize this fact: although there were systems of analyzing the physical movement of dance, for example, Labanotation, Benesh, and Eskhol, there was no tool to probe for meaning in movement. Describing the physical movement in time, space, and effort does not tell us what the movement is about. There were no concepts that could call attention to possibilities of the meaning of the patterned gestures and locomotion in context.

Spheres

Devices	Event	Body in Action	Whole Performance	Discursive Performance	Specific Movement	Intermesh with other Media	Presence
Concretization							
Icon							
Stylization							
Metonym							
Metaphor							
Actualization							

© Judith Lynne Hanna

Figure 9-2 Semantic Grid: Creating and Discovering Meaning in Movement Through Dimensions of Meaning in Dance

In response to this need, I developed a semantic grid (see Figure 9-2; Hanna, 1999 presents the most recent description) to serve as a tool for creating and discovering meaning in movement. The grid, which evolved through the efforts of numerous dancers and researchers attempting to make sense of dances in different parts of the world, represents a broad canvas of possible ways in which dancers embody the imagination. The grid's concepts helped shape my analyses of movement in studies of gender, children and American theater (Hanna, 1983, 1986, 1987, 1988a, 1988b, 1988c/in press, 1989a, 1989b, 1998) and further develop the grid.

Drawing upon semiotic analyses of visual and verbal texts and the variety of dance worldwide, I identified devices and spheres of encoding meaning in movement. In probing meaning, the grid can be imposed on the whole dance and also used to zoom in on smaller units of dance. The grid can help bring into focus informants' verbalizations and researchers' observations and analyses to identify associations of dance with some idea, thing, or emotion.

Dancers may embody the imagination in a single device, in various combinations, or in differing ratios. Dance meaning also may be found in one or more spheres. The researcher can explore whether meaning lies in each cell of the grid, formed by the intersection of the vertical and horizontal lines separating devices and spheres. The cells can be a check-list. Revision and expansion of the grid is expected as it is used to accommodate dance data that do not fall into the proposed categories.

There are at least six symbolic *devices* for conveying meaning that may be utilized in dance. These devices vary in degree of abstraction.

D-1. *Concretization* is movement that reproduces the outward aspect of something. Examples include a dancer depicting a soldier attacking a civilian, a dancer depicting an historical figure such as Hitler, and a wide-open mouth denoting a scream.

D-2. An *icon* represents most characteristics of something and is responded to as if it actually were what it represents. For example, a Haitian dancer manifesting through a specific dance the presence of Ghede, the god of love and death, is treated by fellow Haitians with genuine awe and gender-appropriate behavior—as if he actually were the god himself.

D-3. A *stylization* encompasses conventional and arbitrary gestures or movements. For example, a Western classical ballet *danseur* points to his heart as a sign of love for his lady, and a swing dancer shakes a finger in the Lindy Hop as a sign of joy in moving well.

D-4. *Metonym* is a motional conceptualization of one thing representing another, of which it is a part. An example is an aggressive duet representing a more encompassing battered woman relationship.

D-5. *Metaphor*, the most common way of encoding meaning in dance, involves expressing one thought, experience or phenomenon in terms of another. For example, contrasting movement patterns for men and women can illustrate their distinct biological and social roles, and dancers can perform as animal characters to comment on human behavior. Other examples of metaphor in dance include: performing the dances of another group as a way of identifying with it, being part of it, or even dominating it; mechanical movement symbolizing the rigidity of bureaucracy; dance virtuosity representing human aspiration to transcend the limits of the body.

D-6. *Actualization* is a portrayal of one or several aspects of a dancer's real life. As in verbal speech, dance may reflect a person's actual personality or condition. A dancer who is known to have AIDS can evoke awe during a performance due to this fact.

The devices for encapsulating meaning in dance seem to operate within one or more of seven spheres of communication:

S-1. The dance event itself (e.g., when people attend a dance because it is politically correct),

S-2. The total human body in action (e.g., in a dancer's self-presentation),

S-3. The whole pattern of performance—emphasizing structure, style, feeling, or drama—with the focus on the interrelation of those parts of a dance that give it a distinctiveness, as in a sacred dance,

S-4. The discursive sequence of unfolding movement, including who does what to whom, and how in dramatic episodes (e.g., retelling events of 9-11),

S-5. Specific movements and how they are performed, as when a female parodies a tough male by flexing muscles,

S-6. The intermesh of movements with other communication modes, such as singing, speaking, or costuming (e.g., in the hit Broadway musical *The Lion King*),

S-7. Presence, is the emotional impact of projected sensuality, raw animal quality, or charisma; "the magic of dance," the energy that passes between dancers and to the audience.

Meaning in dance also relies on who does what, when, where, why, how, and with whom. Such variables can help dancers highlight sexual orientation and gender roles. These variables can also help to emphasize ethnic, national, and other group identities which may promote self-esteem and separatism. Cuba's rumba, originally a dance of poor blacks, became the national dance.

Similarly, religions from Christianity to Hinduism have long used dance to convey their precepts and legends of divinity, while in nineteenth century Europe, ballets such as *Swan Lake* and *The Sleeping Beauty* provided ethical, instruction for court and bourgeois behavior. In twentieth century United States, Bill T. Jones's *Last Supper at Uncle Tom's Cabin* called attention to events in American history that should not be repeated. Other issues that would be impolite, politically incorrect, or even treasonous to articulate in verbal language are often expressed (or parodied) through the language of dance. Because dance speaks so powerfully, some religious organizations and totalitarian governments consistently attempt to control it.

Some Further Considerations Concerning Meaning

Dance signifies, as in being a sign of the continuity of the African Ubakala, Igbo lineage, through any of the above devices. However, dance may merely be, for example, continuity in terms of a performer sensing in physical action the quality of continuity. Moreover, dance may be an instrument and effect what continuity signifies. The question of representation of reality lies in the beliefs of viewers or dancers (Hanna, 1987). Even abstract contemporary dance movement that seemingly has no referent beyond itself may refer to other genres of dance and the historical development of dances. In addition, viewers may read meaning into a performance irrespective of a dancer's intention.

Symbolic complexity may involve opposites and inversions, for example, the symbol for love really meaning hate. What appears as concretization may in fact be intended as metaphor. A symbol may have a patent meaning, while the latent meaning may be contained in a constellation of symbols; the contradiction of meaning perhaps corresponding to conflicts. One symbol may have different or condensed meaning; it may be continuously reinterpreted or it may change in intensity over time. The same symbol may have different meanings at different phases in performance. Furthermore, metaphoric equations can operate in two directions at once. Saying the lion is the king of the beasts says something about kings and something about lions. Double metaphors may occur; the representation of an object in turn involves a cultural context or state of affairs. In symbolism there is a range of specificity.

As in the case for verbal language, dance symbols may have synonyms: different images may manifest a single concept. Reincarnation is represented by the Ubakala women's circular, slow, relaxed dance for the birth of a child, as well as the men's angular, rapid, and tense warrior dance. Stylistically similar but situationally different, women's dances for the birth of a child and for a woman's journey to the ancestor world both focus on entry to life stages. Dance symbols may have homonyms, two movements or phrases which look alike in most respects, and neutralization, the phenomenon whereby an opposition or meaning is canceled in a particular context. Dance symbols also involve situational qualifiers of space, time, secularity, and sacredness; the juxtaposition or succession of images; and the sequential occurrence of images to produce a synthesis. There may be cross-channel communication, that is, messages sent in the dance differ from those sent in the accompanying song, music, or costume. The message transmitted and the purpose of the dance may be distinct from each other.

Systems of meaning in dance may be better understood by analyzing them in relation to other meaning systems. A group's general concepts of space, time, energy, mind, and body (which comprise the dance phenomenon) may serve as referents in dance.

Meaning may be deduced through examining how symbolic elements are developed in other aspects of culture. These include cosmology, riddles, proverbs, costume, paraphernalia, music, nondance ritual, myth, polity, economy, social structure, and notions of public and private.

SIGNS OF EMOTION

The communication of emotion—its expression, reading, and feeling—is integral to dance/movement therapy. Appendix 1 presents illustrative emotions. Verbal language is not always the most effective or efficient sign system or discourse to convey the scope, depth, and nuances of ideas, feelings, and things. Cultural teachings help fashion which situations warrant particular expressions (see Thomas, 2001, pp. 157–173). In an ethnographic study of children in a desegregated magnet school (Hanna, 1986, 1988a), I found different patterns between low-income black and middle-income blacks and whites. For example, low-income blacks rolled their eyes, thrust out the lower lip, puffed up their bodies, punched, stomped, and kicked to display anger. Middle-class youngsters, by contrast, were litigious.

Yet, a dance faculty, who asked me to speak on the reciprocity of emotion and movement, reacted with disbelief when I discussed variability in emotional expression. The faculty did not want me to talk about culture and held the position that expression of emotion in dance was universal. Since the body is composed of universal features, and time, space, and energy are universals in human life, some members of the dance, medical, and therapeutic professions erroneously assume that these are experienced in a universal manner. However, assumptions concerning the psychic unity of humans ignore the facts of cultural learning.

Faced with disbelief, I began a study to find out what emotions dance performers intended to convey and what spectators perceived (Hanna, 1983). The setting was two live concert series: the World Explorer Series including Kuchipudi and Kathakali from India, Kabuki from Japan, and various dances from the Philippines. The American Dance Experience Series presented two endangered traditions, black jazz tap and creations of trail-blazing choreographer-performers of modern dance and two avant-garde postmodern performances.

At each concert I interviewed the performers and spoke with some audience members at intermission and after the concert. Because the number of people who could be interviewed was so few, I used a written form to elicit audience members' views on the dance before the first intermission. I chose this part of the concert so that people could have recall and writing time during intermission. The voluntary responses of one-third to one-half of the audiences comprise a nonrandom sample. From a limited sample of dances and respondents, we can conclude that there are different clues to identify the same emotion.

This empirical exploration of the reciprocity of movement and emotion challenged key theorists. Rudolf Laban believed that dance begins in a conception of feeling and expressed actual emotion, whereas Susanne Langer argued the opposite, that emotion was symbolic. Both views have some validity, but there is more. First, emotion may stimulate dance; feeling a particular emotion, a performer expresses it through dancing. Second, emotion may be recalled as a stimulus to dance. Third, the dancer may recall emotion and express it symbolically, rather than actually. Fourth, dancing may induce emotion. Fifth, audience reaction to an ongoing performance may evoke the performer's emotions, which, in turn, affect the dancing. Sixth, however the dancer expresses emotion, the dancer attempts to evoke emotion in the audience.

Even when audience members share a culture, they may offer opposite views on whether or not the dancers conveyed feeling in a dance. Viewing a Douglas Dunn—Deborah Riley duet, forty-six percent of the spectators saw no emotion, while fifty-five percent observed eroticism, a strong emotion. Yet, there are regularities across some cultures (e.g., Moore et al., 1999).

COMPARISON

Comparison is another anthropological tool. Anthropologists who favor minutely contextualized research dismiss comparison. But when we compare and find factors in one dance culture and not in another, we are pushed to ask why. Pursuit of possible answers further advances our quest for understanding dance as human behavior. A comparative perspective suggests the uniqueness of a culture's own dance expression as well as the similarity to others. From a broad overview arise hypotheses of greater generality; formulations that transcend the circumstances of any given case and interpretive insights. Moreover, a comparative perspective is often a mind-stretcher, prejudice-dissolver, and taste-widener.

To compare, it is necessary to impose analytic categories on data in a kind of "deconstruction." Because many groups do not analyze dance, the categories may be ethnocentric, developed largely from a researcher's own traditions, but modified as new knowledge comes to the fore.

Given group diversity and intra-cultural differences, the task of classifying dances presents multiple avenues. Ordinarily, an explicit or implicit theory based on scientific or humanistic concerns underlies the choice of classification scheme. Ultimately, the goal is to formulate general laws that enable us to understand and predict human behavior. To call to the reader's attention some of the complexity of dance in different cultures, Appendix 2 presents a sampling of illustrative kinds of categories, neither all-inclusive nor mutually exclusive.

ASSESSMENT

A recent development in anthropology is evaluation research (Fetterman, 1995a, 1995b, 2000). This is important for dance/movement therapists who want to assess outcomes and evaluate programs for diverse groups. Ethnography can be a useful part of documenting treatment for posttraumatic stress syndrome.

This applied research offers practical direction. For example, investigators can engage in what is called formative assessment, or action research. This means they observe and document what takes place between client and therapist so that therapists can correct problems that are identified. Ongoing evaluation of a dance/movement therapy program and specific practices may disclose problems that practitioners and theorists never knew they had. Such an evaluation may also suggest ways for improvement. It is not sufficient to simply know that a dance/movement therapy program or practice works for it to be replicated; therapists must also understand *how* it works, that is, the process, its pitfalls and how problems are resolved or could be prevented. The steps of self-empowerment evaluation can facilitate transformative learning, that is, the process of reframing reality in ways that facilitate constructive change. A more in-depth description of evaluation research is given by Cruz (Chapter 10) in this text.

NO TRUTH EXISTS

"New" poststructuralist, postcolonialist, and postmodern anthropological methodologies assume an "equality" of groups. These approaches purport to unmask power relations inscribed on the dancing/moving body and to reveal fusions of different dance traditions. Current buzzwords include reflexivity, hegemony, globalization, multiple perspectives and truths, embodiment, writing and rewriting the body. Objectivity and reality are jettisoned as modernist delusions. To counter the postmodern principle that there are no truths, only points of view, anthropologists present various perspectives of members of a culture who often have different pieces of knowledge based on age, gender, sexual orientation, membership in an association, social class, and historical period. Anthropologists often engage in collaborative research in which the perspectives and insights of each team member can challenge the integrity of others. In addition, anthropologists ask for comments on their research findings from the group they study as well as professional colleagues. Note that the September 11, 2001, attacks on the United States challenge the postmodern and postcolonial rejection of ethical judgment and espousal of relativism.

CONCLUSION

American and other societies have become increasingly culturally heterogeneous, and a Western-developed dance/movement therapy has spread to other countries. Consequently, a practice rooted in Western culture may need to make accommodations to work effectively with people of other cultures. Effective therapy requires a practitioner to understand how to communicate with a client from a different culture within the client's concepts of trauma, health and healing, mind, body, emotion, time, space, effort, music, and color. A client's world-view at odds with the theory and method of the therapist creates barriers to healing in addition to placing new stress upon the client (Hanna, 1988c). Here is where anthropological research can make an important contribution.

It can create an awareness of cultural rules for verbal and nonverbal engagement to facilitate negotiating legitimacy and trust in dance/movement therapy. Missteps can impede positive outcomes. Anthropological methods can discover the meaning of movement in context to facilitate communication. Dance/movement therapists may want to explain the process they use in terms of a particular culture's belief system, such as trance and possession, and to draw upon ritual rhythms and movements familiar to the client. Just as contemporary Western medicine is turning to native herbal practices and harnessing their power, so too could dance/movement therapists incorporate native theory and method into their knowledge and practice.

REFERENCES

Acosta, F., Yamamoto, J., & Evans, L. A. (Eds.). (1982). *Effective psychotherapy for low-income and minority patients*. New York: Plenum Press.

Atkinson, D. R., Martin, G., & Sue, D. N. (1989). *Counseling American minorities: A cross-cultural perspective* (3rd ed.). Dubuque, IA: William C. Brown.

Bernard, H. R. (Ed.). (2000). *Handbook of methods in cultural anthropology*. Walnut Creek, CA: Alta Mira Press.

Bernard, H. R. (2001). *Research methods in anthropology: Qualitative and quantitative approaches*. (3rd ed.). Walnut Creek, CA: Alta Mira Press.

Bernstein, B. (1995). Dancing beyond trauma: Women survivors of sexual abuse. In F. J. Levy, with J. P. Fried, & F. Leventhal (Eds.). *Dance and other expressive art therapies: When words are not enough* (pp. 41–58). New York: Routledge.

Boddy, J. (1988). Spirits and selves in North Sudan: The cultural therapeutics of possession and trance. *American Ethnologist, 15*(1), 4–27.

Chang, M., & Leventhal, F. (1995). Mobilizing battered women: A creative step forward. In F. J. Levy, with J. P. Fried, & F. Leventhal (Eds.), *Dance and other expressive art therapies: When words are not enough* (pp. 59–68). New York: Routledge.

Dosamantes-Beaudry, I. (1999). Divergent cultural self construals: Implications for the practice of dance/movement therapy. *Arts in Psychotherapy, 26*(4), 225–231.

Fetterman, D. (1995a). In response. *Evaluation Practice, 16*(2), 179–99.

Fetterman, D. (Ed.) (1995b). *Empowerment evaluation: Knowledge and tools for self- assessment and accountability*. Thousand Oaks, CA: Sage.

Fetterman, D. (2000). *Foundations of empowerment evaluation*. Newbury Park, CA: Sage.

Foner, N. (Ed.). (2001). *Islands in the city: West Indian migration to New York*. Berkeley, CA: University of California Press.

Frank, Z. (1997). Dance and expressive movement therapy: An effective treatment for a sexually abused man. *American Journal of Dance Therapy, 19*(1), 45–61.

Friedson, S. (1996). *Dancing prophets: Musical experience in Tumbuka healing*. Chicago, IL: University of Chicago Press.

Goode, E., & Eakin, E. (2002, September 11). Mental health: The profession tests its limits. *New York Times* (pp. A1, A16–17).

Givens, D. (2002). *The nonverbal dictionary of gestures, signs and body language cues*. Spokane, WA: Center for Nonverbal Studies Press.

Graessner, S., Gurris, N., & Pross, C. (Eds.). (2001). *At the side of torture survivors: Treating a terrible assault on human dignity*. Baltimore, MD: Johns Hopkins University Press.

Gray, A. E. L. (2001). The body remembers: Dance/movement therapy with an adult survivor of torture. *American Journal of Dance Therapy, 23*(1):29–43.

Guindy, H. E., & Schmais, C. (1994). The Zar: An ancient dance of healing. *American Journal of Dance Therapy, 16*(2), 107–120.

Hanna, J. L. (1983). *The performer-audience connection: Emotion to metaphor in dance and society*. Austin and London: University of Texas Press.

Hanna, J. L. (1986). Interethnic communication in children's own dance, play, and protest. In Y. Y. Kim (Ed.). *Interethnic communication* (Vol. 10, *International and intercultural communication annual*) (pp. 176–198). Newbury Park, CA: Sage.

Hanna, J. L. (1987). *To dance is human: A theory of nonverbal communication*. Chicago, IL: University of Chicago Press (Rev. ed.).

Hanna, J. L. (1988a). *Disruptive school behavior: class, race, and culture*. New York: Holmes & Meier.

Hanna, J. L. (1988b). *Dance, sex, and gender: Signs of identity, dominance, defiance, and desire*. Chicago, IL: University of Chicago Press [*Dança, sexo e gênero: Signos de identidade, dominação, desafio e desejo*. Rio de Janeiro, Brazil: Editora Rocco Ltda. 1999].

Hanna, J. L. (1988c/in press). *Dance and stress: resistance, reduction, and euphoria.* New York: AMS Press/*Dance and stress revisited* (Rev. ed.). Lanham, MD: Altamira.

Hanna, J. L. (1989a). African dance frame by frame: Revelation of sex roles through distinctive feature analysis and comments on field research, film, and notation. *Journal of Black Studies, 19*(4), 422–441 (Abstracted in *Cultural Anthropology Methods Newsletter, 1*(2),13, 1989).

Hanna, J. L. (1989b). The anthropology of dance. In L. Y. Overby & J. H. Humphrey (Eds.). *Dance: Current selected research,* I. (pp. 219–237). New York: AMS Press.

Hanna, J. L. (1990). Anthropological perspectives for dance/movement therapy. *American Journal of Dance Therapy, 12*(2), 115–126.

Hanna, J. L. (1995). The power of dance: Health and healing. *Journal of Alternative and Complementary Medicine, 1*(4), 323–327.

Hanna, J. L. (1998, Summer). Undressing the First Amendment and corsetting the striptease dancer. *The Drama Review* (T158), *42*(2), 38–69.

Hanna, J. L. (1999). *Partnering dance and education: Intelligent moves for changing times.* Champaign, IL: Human Kinetics Press (Forthcoming Korean translation: Jungdam).

Hanna, J. L. (2001). The language of dance. *Journal of Health, Physical Education, Recreation and Dance, 72*(4), 40–45, 53.

Hanna, J. L. (2002a, Spring). Reading a universal language? *DCA* (Dance Critics Association) *News,* pp. 6, 15.

Hanna, J. L. (2002b). Lost dance research/found new hubris. *Dance Research Journal, 34*(1), 7–10.

Helman, C. (2000). *Culture, health, and illness* (4th ed.). Boston, MA: Butterworth-Heinemann.

Ho, M. K. (1987). *Family therapy with ethnic minorities.* Newbury Park, CA: Sage.

Jacobs-Huey, L. (2002). Exchange across difference: The production of ethnographic knowledge—the natives are gazing and talking back: Reviewing the problematics of positionality, voice, and accountability among "native" anthropologists. *American Anthropologist, 104*(3), 791–804.

Janzen, J. M. (2002). *The social fabric of health: An introduction to medical anthropology.* Boston, MA: McGraw Hill.

Kleinman, A. (1980). *Patients and healers in the context of culture: An exploration of the borderland between anthropology, medicine, and psychiatry.* Berkeley, CA: University of California Press.

Kleinman, A. (1995). *Writing at the margin: Discourse between anthropology and medicine.* Berkeley, CA: University of California.

Krebs, S. (1975). The film elicitation technique: Using film to elicit conceptual categories of culture. In P. Hockings (Ed.). *Principles of visual anthropology* (pp. 283–302). The Hague: Mouton.

Landy, R. J. (2002). Sifting through the images—a drama therapist's response to the terrorist attacks of September 11, 2001. *The Arts in Psychotherapy, 29,* 135–141.

Layiwola, D. (1999). The problem of literal documentation in African dance studies. Paper presented at Confluences: International Conference on Dance and Music, University of Capetown, South Africa, July 16–19, 1997, p. 7, quoted in E. J. J. Jones, The choreographic notebook: A dynamic documentation of the choreographic process of Kokuma dance theatre, an African-Caribbean dance company. In T.J. Buckland (Ed.). *Dance in the field* (pp. 100-110). London: Macmillan.

Liebmann, M. (Ed.) (1996). *Arts approaches to conflict.* Bristol, PA: Jessica Kingsley.

Madsen, W. (1973). *Mexican-Americans of south Texas* (2nd ed.). New York: Holt, Rinehart & Winston.

McElroy, A., & Townsend, P. K. (1989). *Medical anthropology in ecological perspective* (2nd ed.). Boulder, CO: Westview Press.

Moore, C. C., Romney, A. K., Hsia, T., & Rusch, C. (1999). The universality of the semantic structure of emotion terms: Methods for the study of inter- and intra-cultural variability. *American Anthropologist, 101,* 529–546.

Nichter, M., & Lock, M. (Eds.). (2002). *New horizons in medical anthropology: Essays in honor of Charles Leslie.* New York: Routledge.

Ogbu, J. U., & Simons, H. D. (1998). Voluntary and involuntary minorities: A cultural-ecological theory of school performance with some implication for education. *Anthropology & Education Quarterly, 29*(2), 155–188.

Rubenstein, S. L. (2002). Between terror and terrorists. *AnthroWatch, 10*(1), 3–4.

Salzman, P. C. (2002). On reflexivity. *American Anthropologist, 104*(3), 805–813.

Sebeok, T. A. (2001). *Signs: An introduction to semiotics* (2nd ed.). (Toronto Studies in Semiotics and Communication). Toronto: University of Toronto Press.

Thomas, R. M. (2001). *Folk psychologies across cultures.* Thousand Oaks, CA: Sage.

Zephir, F. (2001). *Trends in ethnic identification among second-generation Haitian immigrants to New York City.* Westport, CT: Bergin and Garvey.

Appendix 1

PARTIAL LIST OF EMOTIONS AND COMMUNICATION DIFFERENCES VARIABLES

	Sender/Expression	*Observer*
	How Physically Expressed–Situation–Qualifier (age, gender) Response	
Anger	Anxiety	Boredom
Competitive	Contempt	Depression
Desire	Disgust	Despair
Ecstasy	Embarrassed	Envy
Eroticism	Fatigue	Fear
Gratitude	Grief	Guilt
Happiness/joy	Hurt	Indignant
Lonely	Nervous	Playful
Pleasure	Pride	Sadness
Shame	Shy	Surprise
Vital	Weak	Withdrawn
Other		

Appendix 2

SAMPLING OF DANCE CATEGORIES
FOR COMPARISON

Catalysts for Dance
    Sacred
        Embodying the supernatural: inner transformation
        Embodying the supernatural: external transformation (masked)
        Representation of divinity
        Health and healing
    Secular
        Representation of deities and spirits as entertainment
        Celebration of event (e.g., birth, death, marriage, harvest, war)
        Education—initiation
        Courtship
        Recreation
        Political action
        Health and healing
        Work
        A special group's dances
    Participation criteria
        Ascription (e.g., age, gender, marital status, social class, political affiliation)
        Achievement (in any domain)
Participation motivation (required, expected, voluntary)
Devices and spheres of encoding/decoding movement used (see Figure 9-2)
Type of music, costume, setting
Pattern of motion (which body parts, locomotion, gestures, and poses used)
Performer-audience interaction (separate, merge, or combination pattern)
Aesthetic criteria
Devices and of encoding/decoding movement
    Concretization; Icon; Stylization; Metonymy; Metaphor; Actualization

Part 4

CREATIVE ALTERNATIVES

AND OPTIONS

Chapter 10

WHAT IS EVALUATION RESEARCH?

ROBYN FLAUM CRUZ

Program evaluation research is a wonderfully pragmatic option for dance/movement therapists to assess aspects of their practice or a particular program of dance/movement therapy (DMT) treatment they institute. Dance/movement therapists can use evaluation findings to convince administrators to keep an existing DMT program, expand it, or even begin a new program in another facility. Many service expansion grants, for example, the Substance Abuse and Mental Health Services Administration's (SAMHSA) Targeted Capacity Expansion grants, require an evaluation plan as part of the grant proposal. When an evaluation has been completed to satisfy such requirements of grant funding, the findings may be used to apply for a continuation of funding or even to apply for new funding. Dance/movement therapists might use evaluation research to effectively expand their services under the auspices of Federal or other types of grants.

Dance/movement therapists who work in agencies accredited by the Joint Commission on Accreditation for Healthcare Organizations (JCAHO) might be familiar with evaluation research in the format of performance improvement projects. Performance improvement projects are mini-evaluations that JCAHO encourages healthcare organizations to use to improve efficiency and service delivery. Evaluation techniques and organizational management techniques are combined in performance improvement projects, with the overall intent of defining and using data to evaluate an organizational intervention.

Evaluation research involves either clearly defining the objectives of the program or practice to be evaluated, or uncovering the issues, concerns, and decisions surrounding it. Often, both of these aspects are incorporated into the evaluation. Evaluation can employ the quantitative and qualitative methods that have been discussed in some detail in this text. But what distinguishes evaluation from other types of research such as quasi-experimental research described in Chapter 3 of this text is its purpose. The purpose of evaluation is to produce findings that assist in making judgments about the merits of a program for informing decision making and policy (Popham, 1972; Borg & Gall, 1983). The purpose of evaluation is quite different from the purpose of research as it is described in other chapters of this volume. In fact, some behavioral scientists do not consider program evaluation to be research (Rose & Fiore, 1999). Yet, excellent evaluation employs the same attention to accountability, validity, and reliability as other forms of research. In addition, evaluation research regularly includes information on the fidelity of the treatment—if the treatment was actually delivered as it was intended—that is sometimes not included in other types of research (Sechrest, West, Phillips, Redner, & Yeaton, 1979).

Evaluations are often used to study a program as an intervention. The impact of the intervention is the focus of the evaluation. In this case, fidelity to the planned intervention is very important to document. The findings of this type of evaluation may be used to improve, continue, or expand the intervention. But the findings can not be used inferentially in the way results of basic or applied research (both experimental and quasi-experimental designs) are used to argue that other populations or settings should benefit from the intervention (Rose & Fiore, 1999). In other words, the primary purpose of research is to develop new knowledge or expand on an existing knowledge base, while program evaluation research provides information that can be used to make decisions about a program.

For evaluation, it is necessary to be very clear and realistic about the goals the program is expected to accomplish and how they should be achieved, even though evaluation does not involve arguments for causation that are central to experimental and quasi-experimental research. The purpose of evaluation is not to demonstrate that changes in participants are attributable to the intervention. Instead, evaluation research is used to demonstrate that the intervention either addressed or failed to address its stated objectives. It is this pragmatic character of evaluation that makes it appealing for expanding DMT programs in many different contexts; evaluation research is applicable to dance/movement therapists who are concerned that research is important for the survival of the profession (Cruz & Hervey, 2001).

ELEMENTS OF PROGRAM EVALUATION

Well-designed evaluations are useful for assessing the effectiveness of programs in achieving program goals. Program goals can include measuring the impact of the program, and this type of goal-oriented evaluation is referred to as *summative* evaluation. Summative evaluations assess the extent to which programs achieve the outcomes described by the program goals. Data should reflect knowledge, attitude, or practice changes and should allow conclusions regarding the overall effectiveness of the program. Evaluation can also be used to strengthen or enhance programs when they are in the early stages of development, and this type of evaluation is referred to as *formative* evaluation. Formative evaluations are conducted to determine the accuracy of program implementation. For example, the consistency of the program, attitudes to the program, or other types of feedback that might be useful in subsequent implementations can be revealed. Evaluation findings can be used to make decisions about whether a program or intervention should be started or continued, or whether a particular program should be chosen when there are multiple alternative programs. For practitioners, evaluation can actually be empowering, by offering a means of documenting the objectives of their work.

For example, an evaluation of dance/movement therapy might be designed to: a) assess whether an organization needs the program; b) describe how the program has been implemented; c) measure outcomes of the program; d) examine the cost effectiveness of the program or compare its cost effectiveness to a similar program with similar objectives; or e) gather information for the purpose of maintaining program quality.

Obviously, these are just a sample of the possible uses of dance/movement therapy program evaluation. Later in this chapter, I present an example of the third possibility mentioned—measuring program outcomes to see if the program objectives were achieved—that illustrates the creative and pragmatic thinking that goes into selecting indicators for evaluation.

Evaluation research studies can use quantitative methods, qualitative methods, or a combination of the two to produce findings. Chapter 3 (Berrol) in this text offers readers in-depth descriptions of quantitative methods, and Chapters 7 (Green) and 8 (Forinash) offer valuable information about qualitative methods. Quantitative data address information such as who, what, how many, or how much. For example, an evaluation of a DMT program with elderly adults in a senior center might note the age, ethnicity, sex, and general health status of the individuals who receive the DMT program. Qualitative data address how and why something is occurring, and for the senior center example, might consist of interviews with the participants about their motivations for attending the DMT program at the center.

Evaluations can be cross-sectional or longitudinal in design, meaning that data can be collected at a single instance to offer a snapshot of the program, or gathered over several time periods to give a more complete view of development or change over time. In many program evaluation studies, data are gathered before the intervention so that comparisons can be made with data at the end of the intervention, similar to a pretest-posttest design in experimental or quasi-experimental research and analogous to the baseline and treatment phases of single-subject design research (see Chapter 6 in this text). Groups that are randomized to interventions or control groups that do not receive the intervention can also be used in evaluation designs. The choice of cross-sectional or longitudinal design and other design features, are determined by the type of evaluation (formative or summative), objectives of the evaluation (impact on learning, behaviors, or other characteristics of participants), and the sources of data that can be arranged.

Often, existing record keeping or documentation provides a source of data, although additional sources may need to be employed or developed specifically for the evaluation. Validity and reliability of measures remain important issues in evaluation research, just as in experimental or quasi-experimental research. An overview of these issues with respect to movement observations often used by dance/movement therapists is given in this text by Cruz and Koch (Chapter 4).

THE PROCESS OF EVALUATION RESEARCH

Planning and conducting evaluation research follows a process similar to that described for a research study in Chapter 3 of this text. The evaluation researcher starts by defining the focus of the evaluation and develops a plan and timetable for the evaluation. To formalize an evaluation, it is important to conduct a review of the literature. Extending the example of evaluating a DMT program at a senior center, the dance/movement therapist might summarize literature that addresses the importance of social contact, psychological changes and needs later in life, and physical activity on the health status of elderly individuals to establish a rationale for the program. The next step is to develop a study design with a description of the evaluation focus or questions. The focus allows the dance/movement therapist to decide if a formative or summative evaluation is appropriate. If the dance/movement therapist is developing the DMT program, a formative evaluation would assist in guiding him or her. If there is an existing program, the therapist might want to gather information on the perceived benefits (if any) of the program to participants. He or she also might want to look at the impact of the program on participants' health status.

Once the focus has been determined, it is necessary to plan what data will be collected and how it will be collected. It is equally important at this stage to plan how the data will be analyzed. Quantitative data can easily be entered into a computer spreadsheet program (such as Microsoft Excel) and summarized in tables that display, for example, how many participants were in the 65- to 69-year-old group and how many were in the 70- to 74-year-old group. Data on the participants' perceptions of the program might be gathered using a survey, but an interview could be used instead to capture perceptions that the dance/movement therapist has not envisioned. The interviews will likely be rather rich, but will be more labor intensive to analyze as each interview will need to be transcribed and coded using a content analysis system that the researcher devises.

Certain aspects of the evaluation are important to include in planning. For example, if the impact of the program is of interest (as is common) it will be vital to keep documentation of the fidelity of the program. Notes on what was done in each session and who participated in each session can be used to produce data on fidelity. If some other group at the senior center, for example, the arts and crafts group, were to be used for comparison purposes it would be important to plan well in advance for collecting data on this group.

Procedures for securing the informed consent of participants and protecting the confidentiality of the program participants are not only needed, but are of the utmost importance. If the senior center had no formal procedures, the dance/movement therapist could contact a research internal review board at a local university or healthcare organization. She or he could also get guidelines from the U.S. Department of Health and Human Services Office of Human Research Protections at: http://ohrp.osophs.dhhs.gov/humansubjects/guidance/45cfr46.htm.

It is possible that many different individuals and groups might have an interest in a dance/movement therapist's evaluation research. For example, the administrative head of the organization, program participants and their families, or local chapters of organizations such as the American Association for Retired People (AARP) might be interested in the DMT program evaluation at the senior center. In evaluation research these interested parties are called stakeholders. It is the responsibility of the evaluation researcher to attend to stakeholders without allowing them to skew or influence the findings of the evaluation.

Once data have been collected and the program as planned is completed, a written report that describes the purpose, methods, findings, and makes recommendations for program improvement completes the evaluation process. Final evaluation research reports have a similar format to research articles. An executive summary (similar to an abstract) gives an overview of the evaluation rationale, plan, and findings. The introduction describes the program, reviews the relevant literature, and gives the purpose of the evaluation. The next section of the report describes the methods used including how data were collected and analyzed. Evaluation findings (similar to research results), a discussion of the findings related to the literature and other relevant program features, and finally recommendations about the program (the real substance of evaluation research) finish the report.

EVALUATION RESEARCH EXAMPLE: PEACE THROUGH DANCE/MOVEMENT: A VIOLENCE PREVENTION PROGRAM

Social worker and dance/movement therapist Lynn Koshland developed a program using DMT to address aggression and violent behaviors of young, school-aged children. The actual development of the program took place over a period of several years as she attempted to address the needs of one of the public schools in which she worked. While there appeared to be benefits of the program for children in the school, Lynn, the principal, and the school district administrators were interested in using the program in other schools and desired more direct information about its impact. Using grant funds from the Marian Chace Foundation of the American Dance Therapy Association, Lynn has completed an evaluation of the program that serves as an excellent example of evaluation research.

The program, Peace Through Dance/Movement, used a dance/movement therapy group process that focused on socialization and engagement of children in a creative, problem-solving experience using children's stories and movement. The program included two components, a weekly session with the children, and the introduction of classroom interventions that the teachers and children learned and used to reinforce parts of the program. Lynn worked with the natural situation in the school, where there was growing concern about aggressive behaviors with the lower grades, and she was asked to offer her program to three first-grade classes, two second-grade classes, and two third-grade classes. She delivered the program to five of these groups and an expressive arts therapy staff person trained by Lynn delivered the program to the other two groups. The program was planned as twelve weekly sessions fifty minutes in length in which teachers participated and learned the classroom interventions, consisting of chants and hand gestures, along with the children.

Several sources were identified for gathering data about the effectiveness of the program. The children provided one source, and due to their ages, a picture-based assessment (Goldstein, 1999) was selected and revised slightly to record their perceptions of: a) aggressive incidents that they saw at school; b) where the incidents took place at school; c) feelings about witnessing the incidents; and d) how children handled themselves when they saw the incidents. Baseline data before the intervention was begun were collected and perceptions after the intervention was completed were also collected. Qualitative data were obtained from the children via group interviews at the end of the program, as well as from detailed session notes that were taken during the intervention. These data provided more information about the children's perspectives on what was helpful, fun, or different about the program.

Teachers provided another source of information and they completed an assessment form for each child in their classroom, a checklist of behaviors, both at baseline and completion of the intervention. Two different forms of the checklist were used, one at baseline and one at the conclusion of the program, to address issues of teachers' response biases. For example, teachers might remember how they scored a child previously and repeat that score or deviate from it purposely rather than in response to the child's actual behaviors at the time rated. Both checklists asked teachers to rate aggressive and pro-social behaviors.

The principal provided a third source of information as aggressive incidents required reporting to the principal, and she kept a log of each incident and the specific classroom in which the incident took place. Finally, Lynn employed a staff member to make random observations of the classrooms involved in the program intervention to note aggressive and prosocial behaviors using a checklist devised for this purpose and also noting the teachers' use of the classroom interventions that were planned to help generalization of the program. Using multiple sources of data in this way strengthened the evidence about the program, and in addition, the data from the principal allowed comparisons to classrooms that did not receive the intervention so that a control group type of design was possible for this data source.

This was a strong evaluation design because of several factors that should be pointed out. There were multiple informants or sources of data, a pretest-posttest design was used for some data sources, comparison group data were used for one data source, and quantitative and qualitative data provided information spanning the range of what was needed—who, what, how much, how and why. For example, the results were able to show that a quantitative change took place in the children's perceptions of aggressive acts they witnessed, but in addition, their comments about the program helped to explain why and how the children experienced these changes. Using observation and ratings scales that included noting pro-social behaviors as well as aggressive behaviors, allowed Lynn to see if the program not only decreased aggressive behaviors but also promoted pro-social behaviors with the children.

Because quantitative measures were used for the children's and teachers' perceptions of aggressive behaviors, the evaluation findings include the results of statistical tests applied to the data. In reporting these results, statistically significant findings for teachers included noted decreases in children instigating fights, failing to calm down, being short tempered and quick to show anger, being aggravated or abusive when frustrated, being involved in physical fights, throwing articles, and damaging school property. Significant decreases noted by students included seeing or experiencing arguing, someone doing something wrong, and someone throwing something. The classroom observations showed a significant decrease in the frequency of negative behaviors. No difference in pro-social behaviors was noted. As Lynn summarized the findings (Koshland, in preparation),

> The results revealed statistically significant decreases in aggression and problem behaviors that the teachers noticed; a decrease of aggression both seen and experienced by students; and a significant difference in the incidents reported to the principal's office for classrooms that attended the program compared to classrooms that did not attend. In addition, random classroom observations also showed a decrease of problem behaviors (p. 27).

Figure 10-1 displays the numbers of incidents reported to the principal for the children in the program and those in classrooms that did not par-

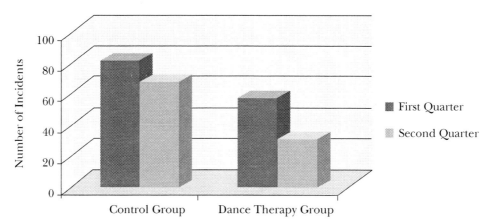

Figure 10-1   Rates of Incidents of Aggression Reported to the Principal's Office Before Program (First Quarter) and after Program Intervention (Second Quarter)

ticipate before the program and after its completion. Incidents for the program group decreased significantly compared to the classrooms that did not receive the program. While both groups showed a decrease in incidents, the decrease for the Peace Through Dance/Movement children was statistically greater than for the other classrooms. Lynn used this graph in her final report to the school district (Koshland, 2003).

As a result of this evaluation, Lynn gained support from both the school district and the principal for continuing the program. She was also asked to present the program to other schools in the district, and to expanding the program for older children. She plans to continue evaluating the program and to further explore ideas and observations generated from this initial evaluation about how the program works. She summarized this as:

> It is significant to note that when children can explore many different ways of self-control within a large group, and increase their focus of those aspects that require paying attention to, and ignoring those aspects which interfere with learning (i.e., joining negative behaviors) while being introduced to pro-social behaviors, a practice playground environment is created that allows a safe contained space for applying less aggressive ways (Koshland, in preparation, pp. 27-28).

CONCLUDING REMARKS

Sechrest et al. (1979) addressed some neglected problems in evaluation research that they termed the strength and integrity of treatments. They argued that because treatments delivered in real settings are "rarely standardized, often complex, can be delivered by poorly trained or unmotivated people, or can be disrupted by events in the treatment context—evaluation research may fail to find a significant effect" (p. 15). This is important because it causes the evaluation research to fail to inform the stakeholders of what the effect might be if the treatment had been delivered as planned. This issue of fidelity was introduced earlier in this chapter, but is of such importance that it is worth mentioning again. In the DMT evaluation example described, Lynn Koshland addressed this problem by training a carefully chosen individual to assist in delivering the program, and by planning the program elements sufficiently in advance that it was possible to train someone else to use the program.

Strength as used by Sechrest et al. (1979) is the planned intensity with which the treatment is intended to be delivered, and this is an important element not only of evaluation research but of all research that investigates a treatment intervention. How much of the intervention is actually needed to produce a discernable effect on the participants? Are two DMT sessions per week enough to produce an effect in six weeks? Are two insufficient, but three enough? There are obviously no clear answers to these questions, and this is certainly a topic for DMT research to tackle—what is the dose of DMT needed to produce change? In the Peace Through Dance/Movement project, this issue was partially addressed by introducing classroom interventions (chants and gestures) that teachers and children learned and practiced together to maintain and encourage self-control. These interventions provide one way of conceptualizing strengthening the dose of a program; they served to remind the children of the sessions and what they experienced and learned in the program, while generalizing those skills to a new environment. As more dance/movement therapists engage in evaluation research, I have no doubt that other creative solutions will be generated.

Before concluding this brief introduction to evaluation research, a close relative of evaluation research should be mentioned. Action research is a form of evaluation research that can be very useful to dance/movement therapists. Jill Green also describes action research in this text (Chapter 7).

Because therapy is a process, it can be difficult to evaluate. Dance/movement therapists are trained to assess and treat clients, but are not trained in how to evaluate their own work or the possibilities for involving their clients in this process. Yet, evaluating what dance/movement therapists do in systematic ways can truly inform individuals about their practices in addition to supporting their employment. Action research is a broadly used term in education that refers to a participatory approach to evaluation (Stringer, 1999). While action research has been used with communities and groups, it can also be applied to clinical work to enhance and develop practice, and to address specific questions or problems. It can be as simple as reviewing goals and procedures, and the extent to which objectives are achieved. It can involve clients and other staff as co-researchers, and be as elementary or complex as one chooses to make it. Core elements of this type of research are to establish a formal process for exploring a question or issue by defining it, involving key informants and information sources, and analyzing component parts via critical thinking, planning, implementing, and evaluating strategies. Using these techniques can involve simple activities like the therapist posing a question to himself or herself and a client, "How will we know when participating in dance/movement therapy has helped you?" Or, "What do you expect dance/movement therapy to help you accomplish?" It can be as complex as discovering how the dance/movement therapy program functions within an organization. Possible uses for this type of research can range from enriching the therapist's experience to providing a structure for supervision, or even producing a published paper.

Evaluation research holds rich opportunities for dance/movement therapists and the profession. It can be used to create evidence and arguments to start and expand DMT services and to examine important questions related to one's practice. While challenging, evaluation does not require the rigor of experimental or other types of research that are used to increase knowledge with the purpose of generalizing to other populations and settings. Instead, evaluation research offers a pragmatic way of examining DMT programs and extending practice through creating opportunities for dance/movement therapists. In this way, it provides a means by which dance/movement therapists can use their work to positively guide the profession.

REFERENCES

Borg, W. R., & Gall, M. D. (1983). *Educational research: An introduction* (4th ed.). New York: Longman.

Cruz, R. F., & Hervey, L. W. (2001). The American Dance Therapy Association research survey. *American Journal of Dance Therapy, 23*(2), 89–118.

Department of Health and Human Services. (2001, November 13). *Code of Federal Regulations Title 45 Public Welfare Department of Health and Human Services National Institutes of Health Office for Protection from Research Risks Part 46 Protection of Human Subjects*. Retrieved October 27, 2003, from http://ohrp.osophs.dhhs.gov/humansubjects/guidance/45cfr46.htm.

Goldstein, A. P. (1999). *Low level aggression: First steps on the ladder to violence*. Chicago, IL: Research Press.

Koshland, L. (2003). *School district report for research pilot study at Edison Elementary School*. Unpublished manuscript.

Koshland, L. (in preparation). *Evaluating a multicultural dance/movement therapy violence prevention program*. Unpublished manuscript.

Popham, W. J. (1972). *An evaluation guidebook: A set of practical guidelines for the educational evaluator*. Los Angeles, CA: The Instructional Objectives Exchange.

Rose, D. S., & Fiore, K. E. (1999). Practical considerations and alternative research methods for evaluating HR programs. *Journal of Business and Psychology, 14*(2), 235–251.

Sechrest, L., West, S. G., Phillips, M. A., Redner, R., & Yeaton, W. (1979). Some neglected problems in evaluation research: Strength and integrity of treatments. In L. Sechrest, S. West, M. Phillips, R. Redner, and W. Yeaton (Eds.). *Evaluation Studies Review Annual* (pp. 15–35). Beverly Hills, CA: Sage.

Stringer, E. T. (1999). *Action research*. (2nd ed.) Thousand Oaks, CA: Sage.

Chapter 11

ARTISTIC INQUIRY IN DANCE/MOVEMENT THERAPY

LENORE WADSWORTH HERVEY

INTRODUCTION

With every dance/movement therapy thesis I witness coming into the world, I am impressed again with the natural, if unexpected, connection between research and creativity, art, and aesthetics. It has been my job for many years to serve as midwife to students and their theses, and once I realized that research was facilitated by many of the same experiences as the creative process, research became easier for my students and me. Furthermore, when we recognized that our dance/movement therapy skills could be used to gather and analyze data, and our artistic skills could assist in presenting findings, research became a more authentic reflection of our clinical and artistic practices. Most subtly, when we understood that our aesthetic values influenced the form taken by the research design and finished product, research became more rewarding.

I recently described in greater depth than is possible here, artistic inquiry as an alternative, arts-based form of research that could utilize a range of skills already familiar to many dance/movement therapists (Hervey, 2000), and I refer interested readers to that work. In this chapter of *Dance/Movement Therapists In Action* I will offer a more concise portrayal of this method, which like the creative process, is impossible to prescribe. To assist this discussion, one complete actual research project and several brief hypothetical ones that richly illustrate artistic inquiry in dance/movement therapy will provide an inside glimpse of how the process may unfold.

ARTISTIC INQUIRY AS A RESEARCH METHOD

The ideas behind artistic inquiry are not new, and are in fact older than the scientific method, which is a relatively new emergence in intellectual history. Simultaneous to the past 300 years of growing enthusiasm about positivist science and its successful application to many fields of study, scholars have provided reminders that logical, analytic methods of reasoning are not the only ways to understand experience or phenomena. Philosophers from Berkeley and Hume in the eighteenth century to Kuhn, Gadamer and Barzun in the twentieth remind us that the dominant paradigm is not the only paradigm. Understanding much of human experience, including art and creativity, requires ways of knowing that can best be described as aesthetic, emotional, and intuitive. Many have asserted that study in the human sciences needs an epistemological approach that is independent of the scientific method (Gadamer, 1998).

More recently, educational researchers like Elliot Eisner (1991, 1995, 1997) have proposed research methods based on artistic experience, as has expressive arts therapist Shaun McNiff (1987, 1993, 1998). Their descriptions of these methods include the following characteristics in common with *qualitative* methods and distinct from more traditional, *quantitative* methods such as experiments and surveys.

1. "Respect for the emergence of meaning as a result of a relationship between researcher and the phenomena under consideration" (McNiff, 1987, p. 282).
2. A focus not on prediction or control, but rather on understanding through indwelling and empathy (Eisner, 1997).
3. Consistency with the values and methods of the profession (McNiff, 1993).
4. "The major instrument is the investigator himself" (Eisner, 1997, p. 8).
5. Emotion as central to knowing (Eisner, 1997).
6. "Grounded upon a comprehensive and systematic integration of empirical [sense-based] and introspective methods" (McNiff, 1998, p. 50).

Features of arts-based research that distinguish it further from other *qualitative* methods include:

1. "The smell of the studio," staying "close to the practice of art and the statements of artists," respecting images, and allowing the artists to present themselves authentically (McNiff, 1987, p. 291).
2. The use of "an evocative form whose meaning is embodied in the shape expressed" (Eisner, 1991, p. 6). Freedom from linearity through image, poetic expression, narrative, dialogue, et cetera (McNiff, 1987). The use of expressive language (or images) (Barone & Eisner, 1997).
3. Validity determined by the persuasiveness of the vision of the artist (Eisner, 1991) or the creation of a believable "virtual reality" (Barone & Eisner, 1997).
4. The presence of ambiguity (Barone & Eisner, 1997).
5. "Trust in the intelligence of the creative process and a desire for relationships with the images that emerge from it" (McNiff, 1998, p. 37).

6. "Final studies [that] are distinctly individuated expressions, more likely to be different from one another than similar" (McNiff, 1998, p. 38).

A research method, such as artistic inquiry, is a coherent set of procedures appropriate to the research question, the research context and subjects, and the researcher's skills and philosophy. In practice, research designs, especially within the qualitative paradigm, rarely reflect the pure method as described by research theoreticians. Many researchers borrow aspects of one method or another to construct a design that best suites the needs of their research endeavor. For instance a quasi-experimental design may have developmental characteristics. Evaluation research may gather both qualitative and quantitative data. A community-based action research project may have an artistic outcome, such as a theatrical presentation. So when considering artistic inquiry, the degree to which a research project meets some definitive criteria only helps distinguish it to a greater or lesser extent from other methods. It too, is rarely found in a pure form. Artistic inquiry, like any research, is a focused, systematic inquiry with the purpose of contributing to a useful body of knowledge. In addition it will have some or all of the following characteristics:

1. It uses artistic methods of data collection, data analysis, and/or presentation of findings.
2. It engages in and acknowledges a creative research process.
3. It is motivated and determined, at least in part, by the aesthetic values of the researcher(s).

While examining each of the three criteria identified above it will become clear how they not only suggest unique research techniques or tools, but also reflect ideas, skills, methods, and values that are central to dance/movement therapy.

Throughout this chapter, examples will be provided in which the researcher is also the therapist, and the research subjects are also therapy clients. This is not to suggest that artistic inquiry need be exclusively clinically based. Rather it is hoped that these vignettes will depict research appropriate to clinical contexts, and will support the image of dance/movement therapists as researchers. However, it is essential to keep in mind the distinction between *therapeutic* goals and methods, and *research* questions and methods. Although a therapist may be engaging in research about the therapy process, the research must be conceptualized separately, with independent questions, goals, and procedures. The clients' needs must not be overshadowed by the researchers' needs. For ethical reasons, in all cases when therapist and researcher are the same person, and when client and subject are the same person, the goals and outcomes of the therapy must take priority over the goals of the research. All aspects of ethical practice of research and therapy must be considered when engaging clients in any kind of research, artistic inquiry not withstanding.

In some therapeutic relationships it may be appropriate for the client(s) to be actively engaged in addressing a research question of interest to both the therapist and the client(s). In cases such as these, the clients may be considered *co-researchers* and may participate in as much of the research design, data collection, data analysis, and presentation of findings as possible, while still addressing their therapeutic goals. The feasibility of this kind of collaboration increases when the therapeutic goals are a psycho/social skill set that includes cooperation, empowerment, creativity, self-esteem, relationship building, community action, assertiveness, et cetera. Care must be taken not to involve clients in activities that compromise essential aspects of the therapeutic relationship, such as trust, emotional safety, and confidentiality. The co-researcher relationship is not unique to artistic inquiry, but evolved out of the qualitative paradigm's recognition of the value of all research participants' experiences (Reason & Rowan, 1981).

ARTISTIC INQUIRY USES ARTISTIC METHODS
OF DATA COLLECTION, DATA ANALYSIS,
AND/OR PRESENTATION OF FINDINGS

By "artistic methods" I mean art-making. The art-making in which dance/movement therapists most often participate and are most skilled is dance. They are also especially skilled at helping untrained dancers make dances. Therefore some form of dance-making could be central to the research process. What would dance-making as data collection, and dance-making as data analysis, entail? How might the dance that is made be used to present findings?

In any research project, data must be collected, then analyzed, and then the findings of the analysis must be organized and presented in an appropriate form. Imagine that the research question is: What are Hispanic immigrant clients' experiences of acculturation and how are they expressed in a culturally diverse dance/movement therapy group? (Jimenez-Figueroa, 2003). There are certainly many ways to find answers to this compound question, but a dance/movement therapist could ask her clients or co-researchers to answer it through movement and dance. One form of the research question might be framed for the participants simply as "Show me how you feel when you are the only Hispanic person in the group." Another way the therapist could ask might be, "Show me with your hands how it feels to speak English," or "Show me how far away you feel from your culture today." The data received might then come in the form of gestures, body shapes, spatial relationships, and facial expressions.

One of the challenges of dance as a form of data collection is that it is transient, as any dancer or choreographer knows. In order to use dance as data, it must be captured in some way, so that it can be looked back upon (or re-searched) in order to be analyzed. How can a client's movement response to a research question be preserved, to be looked at again?

The most obvious way to preserve movement is video recording, which can be conveniently reviewed and analyzed in any number of ways. Confidentiality is of course a concern, and whenever video recordings are made of clients or subjects, written informed consent must be obtained and kept on file by the researcher. The therapist/researcher must also be sensitive to the effects that the presence of a video camera might have on the therapeutic process.

Laban Movement Analysis and the Kestenberg Movement Profile are two movement analysis methods in which many dance/movement therapists are trained. Each can provide in-depth description about the nature of an individual's selected movements or about his or her complete movement repertoire, or profile. Being able to thoroughly document a person's movement style with depth and accuracy is one way to preserve and assist in recalling his or her movement qualities for further examination.

Two other readily available methods to gather movement as data are the dancers' and choreographers' tools of repetition and memorization. Client and researcher can participate together in repeating and committing a movement to memory. Thus the first step is taken toward transforming a collection of movement data into a dance/movement vocabulary that can then be revisited, shared with others, added to over time, and understood more deeply with every repetition.

Perhaps the way dance/movement therapists most regularly collect movement data is by embodying selected qualities of client movement in a method known as *kinesthetic empathy* or *kinesthetic attunement*. With accurate reflection, the process of data analysis begins through the efforts of the researcher/therapist to understand the movement and its message. This movement intervention has two primary *therapeutic* functions. The first is that the client, consciously or unconsciously, feels accurately seen. (In cases where literal reflection or mirroring of movement is therapeutically appropriate, a simple question to the client, such as "Like this?" can confirm the accuracy of the therapist/researcher's perception and potentially engage the client more actively in the therapy or the research.) The second therapeutic function, which can also be part of the data analysis, is that in accurate attunement, reflection, or mirroring, the therapist learns something important about the client. He or she learns on a kinesthetic, emotional, and intuitive level how it feels to be in that movement, expressing that particular feeling or image, in that particular body. When this information is felt deeply and known tacitly in the body, it may not always be possible to articulate fully in words, but it can still be useful information to the therapy and to an artistic inquiry.

Another dance/movement therapy method that can be used as a form of data collection and analysis is *somatic countertransference* (Lewis, 1984). When a therapist works with a client in an embodied manner, moving together, attuning, witnessing, or reflecting movement, he or she may experience impulses to move, sensations in the body, and/or images in response to the client's unconscious material. Many dance/movement therapists are trained to use these images and sensations as a source of information about the client, leading to greater understanding of the client's experience and therapeutic issues. If we consider the client's dance/movement and the therapist's somatic countertransference as part of the research data, then the further exploration of these can be understood as part of the data analysis, and the information gathered as a result can be seen as findings of the analysis.

For example, imagine that the therapist/researcher who is working with the group of Hispanic immigrants in this example is a Caucasian, Euro-American woman of privileged socio-economic status. As she facilitates, moves with, and witnesses her clients'/co-researchers' responses to the research questions about their experiences of acculturation, she becomes aware of feeling guilty and ashamed in her body, and wanting to retreat from the movement experience. In her role as therapist, this is potentially important countertransference information or data. Similarly, in her role as researcher, this may alert her to unconscious information embedded in her co-researchers' answers to the research question. To understand its meaning further, the therapist/researcher enters into further analysis of the data by embodying this guilt and shame, and inviting movement dialogue with the clients/co-researchers. The dialogue could lead to awareness on the part of the clients/co-researchers of projection and blame unconsciously placed on the therapist for the hardships experienced during acculturation. This discovery then becomes part of the findings of the analysis.

With the meaning that can be revealed through analyzing the somatic countertransference, in addition to videotapes of the sessions, and a collection of recalled movements, the researcher/therapist and clients could engage in a creative process of dance-making that further analyzes the research data. Dance-making in the service of research must remain committed to the genuine movement data as the primary creative resource for the choreography. As will be illustrated in the example later in this chapter, it may be tempting for the artist/researcher to abandon the original movement data in order to create an aesthetically pleasing work of art. If this occurs, the authenticity of the data will be lost, and the credibility, and therefore the value, of the research will be compromised.

Making a dance, as many readers will know, involves an examination and re-examination of each movement, each association, each image evoked, until a sequence of movements is discovered that most accurately and effectively communicates the intended meaning. This intensive checking and re-checking through dialogue with the movement, in order to refine and manifest meaning is analogous to data analysis procedures used in other qualitative methodologies (Strauss & Corbin, 1990; Moustakas, 1990; Janesick, 1994; Oldfather & West, 1994; Stinson, 1995). In the example imagined here, the completed dance might seek to express the feelings carried around in the body in relation to those seen as more powerful members of the dominant cultural majority. There might also be a role in the dance for someone who can embody the feelings of shame and guilt of majority cultural group members.

If we understand dance-making as data analysis, then it is easy to see performance as presentation of findings. If clients are involved in performance, they must be given absolute control to determine the right audiences and venues so as not to endanger through inappropriate or unsafe exposure the therapeutic gains made. Venue options could range from an informal performance for clients in their usual meeting place to presentations for friends and family at home or church; for agency staff and administrators in community space; for the therapist's colleagues at a conference; or for the public on a theatrical stage. With the written consent of clients, video-recorded performances can also expand the audience possibilities. Performance can be frightening and/or empowering, and once again, the therapeutic goals must take priority over the research goals. With careful and thoughtful preparation, both goals may be achieved.

Although I have described artistic inquiry as it might unfold using dance, any medium in which the therapist/researcher or clients/subjects feel competent may be used to enhance the collection and analysis of data, and the presentation of findings. Multimedia presentations are often the most powerful communicators. Readers may want to refer to Shaun McNiff's comprehensive work, *Art-based Research* (1998), for further guidance in using art images and media in research.

ARTISTIC INQUIRY ENGAGES IN AND ACKNOWLEDGES THE CREATIVE PROCESS

The descriptive research about creativity is rich with narratives from researchers in many fields who have described creative processes that are essential to their work. Albert Einstein acknowledged that during research, visual, kinesthetic, and intuitive nonverbal processes were active at his most creative moments (Braud & Anderson, 1998). The mathematician Poincare (1908/1952) recounted a prolonged conscious struggle with a mathematical problem, finally resolved by an unpredictable and sudden illumination from his unconscious. Physicist Richard Feynman (1985/1997) discovered the importance of play in facilitating the flow of his research ideas. More recently, authors Denise Shekerjian and Poe Bronson both described their research interviewing and analysis in terms that resonate with the creative process. There were the "untidiness and inconsistency" of a "nonlinear phenomenon," themes that "separated and floated to the surface like cream" (Shekerjian, 1990, pp. xxii–xxiii), and "a blind winding road" leading to the conclusion that "the human soul resists taxonomy" (Bronson, 2002, p. xix). Perhaps because their experiences seem so private and subjective, researchers rarely include them as a part of their research methodologies. Maybe because these aspects of the process seem impossible to predict and replicate, they don't have methodological value to other researchers within scientific fields.

In contrast, artistic inquiry acknowledges the creative process of the research. Rigorous self-observation and reflexive explication of the creative process are required as part of the method. Because dance/movement therapy is so intrinsically dependent upon the creative processes of both the therapist and the client, artistic inquiry seems well suited. Therapists, choreographers, and others who have committed themselves to extended creative projects know that the process is not linear, predictable, or replicable. It seems to require expecting the unexpected, appreciating paradox, and having patience for the unknown. The artistic inquiry process has the same qualities, as well as patterns like those that have been recognized by researchers of the creative process (Moustakas, 1990; Nachmanovitch, 1990; Shekerjian, 1990; Wallas, 1926). The creative process can be thought of as having several phases that do not follow one another in a linear fashion, but proceed cyclically and simultaneously, moving toward transformation of raw data into finished product. To illustrate the parallels between the creative and research processes, these phases can be described in terms common to both.

Data Gathering Phase

Aesthetic or intellectual curiosity, inspiration, passion, frustration, requirement, or even desperation can motivate the formulation of a question that focuses the inquiry. The search can include both consciously directed exploration and less-than-conscious meanderings. It most definitely requires a thorough literature/media review, followed by various modes of data collection such as verbal, written, or movement interviews; video-recording movement; individual or group improvisation on the research question; discussions; intensive observation; historical research; reflective journaling in writing or other art media; et cetera. This goes on until saturation has been achieved. Two common signs of conscious and unconscious saturation, respectively, are encountering the same data repeatedly and dreaming about the data.

Inner Dialogue or Data Analysis Phase

The artist/therapist/researcher attempts to come to an understanding of the data through some sort of analysis. This is the most difficult process to describe in artistic inquiry, as it often requires taking the data deeply into the self and listening for the meaning that will be revealed. In action this might look like repetitive exposure and intensive improvisation with the data in movement, words, or images. Some examples of data analysis methods were given in the previous section on artistic methods of data analysis. The analysis culminates in a transformation of the raw data into a new form that synthesizes and expresses its themes, patterns, messages, or essences.

Expression or Presentation of Results

The form is shared, in progressive stages of completeness, with co-researchers, peers, advisors, internal review boards, committees, and audiences. The presentation venues could include advisement meetings, consultations, in-services, conferences, rehearsals, and/or performances.

Outer Dialogue or Regulating Feedback

Each sharing event stimulates questions, confirmation, challenges, and recommendations that can be incorporated into multiple revisions and repetitions. This refining and regulating sends the artist/researcher back into multiple cycles of the creative process, resulting in a final product that is accepted by the intended audience.

ARTISTIC INQUIRY IS MOTIVATED AND DETERMINED BY THE AESTHETIC VALUES OF THE RESEARCHER(S)

In its most common usage, the term "aesthetics" typically refers to a culture's definition and determination of beauty, or to the branch of philosophy that studies such things. A description of aesthetics I find most helpful in relation to research in dance/movement therapy is *the guiding set of values that determine one's appreciation of qualities reflected in form*. In order to understand this definition and the part aesthetics plays in artistic inquiry, three concepts need to be addressed more fully: qualities, appreciation, and form. I will refer to our example of the Hispanic co-researchers' experiences of acculturation to illustrate.

Qualities

More than simply the surface characteristics or features of a thing, qualities are the perceivable manifestations of its essential nature. A commonly used example of this is the *appleness* of an apple, or the qualities that distinguish it from other fruits. An apple is crunchy, sweet yet tart, juicy, round, red, et cetera. Imagine the qualities that might make one of our Hispanic immigrant co-researchers uniquely who she or he is, like courage, flexibility, fearfulness, or familial loyalty. Imagine the qualities that make an experience, such as acculturation, uniquely what it is. Imagine finally the specific qualities of movement that might reflect this person's experience and how those might be presented in the research findings.

Appreciation

The dictionary provides several definitions of "appreciate," each of which adds dimension to our discussion (*Webster's New Collegiate*, 1981, p. 55). Imagine using each kind of appreciation while creating a dance and selecting *which* sequence of movements most effectively expresses what clients/co-researchers have shared about their experience of acculturation.

1. To grasp the nature, worth, quality or significance of.
2. To value or admire highly.
3. To judge with heightened perception or understanding: be fully aware of.

From the infinite fields of movement, costumes, music, set designs, dancers, and venues researchers must use their aesthetic appreciation to guide them in selecting the best options to express their intended meaning.

Form

"The unique configuration of the qualities of a thing determines its form. How its qualities are arranged in space and time in relation to each other make the form exist" (Hervey, 2000, pp. 72–73). The manifestation and arrangement of our Hispanic immigrant co-researcher's personal qualities, the qualities of their experience, and the movement qualities that express that experience, into a dance in time and space are the form the research presentation might take.

It may seem obvious that artists have aesthetic sensibilities that guide their actions toward creating "good" artistic work. Likewise, every culture has an aesthetic, as does every school or period of art, that reflects its values regarding goodness, beauty, and even health. Perhaps it is less evident that every person has a culturally influenced set of aesthetic values that guide many of his or her decisions, such as decorating a home, buying a gift, getting dressed, or selecting a mate. The ways we move are also determined to an extent by the aesthetics of our cultures.

Does it seem reasonable, then, that different professions might have unique guiding sets of values that determine their members' selection and creation of forms relevant to their work, that reflect qualities they find valuable? Consider what forms dance/movement therapists are concerned with: the body and movement obviously, but also work spaces, movement assessments, DMT sessions, professional presentations, and more. What qualities might dance/movement therapists prefer in these forms that other professionals might not perceive or care about? Is it possible to imagine how forms of research within dance/movement therapy might also reflect professional aesthetic values?

Research methods are in part determined by the aesthetic of the group, profession, and/or culture that is served by that research. Research conducted within the scientific community produces forms with aesthetic qualities that reflect logical order, systematic analysis, and linear visual display. For example, one would not expect to hear music as a display of the results of a scientific study. Although it might be possible, the choice of form would not be congruent with the aesthetic of the scientific method. Professional journals uphold a particular aesthetic as well, as evidenced by writing style and format, page layout, cover, graphics, and choice of font.

If dance/movement therapists were given complete freedom to determine the forms that their research processes and products would take, what would they look like? This is the question that artistic inquiry invites dance therapists to answer. In practice, it generates questions such as these:

What would the place look like where the information was shared with the selected audience? Would it be a stage that imitated life? A neutral abstraction? A natural setting? The actual context in which therapist and client work together?

Where would the audience be in relation to the work shared? How long would it take? What sounds and lighting would accompany it to heighten the experiential understanding of the audience?

If presented in a repeatable, static form, what medium would be used? Book, paper, audio, video, digital, clay? If people were to perform the findings, who would they be? What would they do? How would they look? How would they sound? How would they interact with one another and the audience?

These are the aesthetic choices of artists, permitted entry into the realm of research by artistic inquiry.

WHY CHOOSE ARTISTIC INQUIRY?

The Nature of the Research Topic, Context, and Data

When a topic has not yet been researched sufficiently to develop a hypothesis, then more data of descriptive, qualitative, or artistic nature are needed before it is possible to use a scientific experimental method of investigation. If the data is embedded in a context that cannot be manipulated without altering the essential nature of the experience and the information it yields, then again, some form of qualitative inquiry would be best suited.

If the research is about inner experiences of clients or therapists, and if the resulting data is expected to be rich in emotional, intuitive, imaginal, or embodied content, then artistic inquiry that can transform this raw data into communicable artistic form without losing its authenticity is the best approach. Additionally, artistic inquiry would be the ideal method if the research subjects are motivated to create a dance performance or other artistic event or product to share with a particular audience.

The Researcher(s)

The success of artistic inquiry depends largely on the abilities of the artist/researcher. If the inquiry is to be conducted in dance/movement, then the necessary research skills include accurate kinesthetic attunement, sufficient dance technique, strong observation skills, and creativity, especially in the forms of improvisation and choreography. If nonprofessional co-researchers are involved, then commitment to participation, sufficient time to contribute to the process, cooperation, and informed consent are necessary from them as well.

DETERMINING TRUTH AND VALUE

Put simply, validity criteria are used to determine whether a study's findings are true, and whether they will be of value to consumers. However, truth and value are among some of humanity's most complex ideas, and so the multiple criteria for determining them reflect this complexity, and are beyond the scope of this chapter to fully describe. Researchers within the qualitative paradigm have developed methods of determining validity that are consistent with the particular complexity and philosophy of qualitative inquiry. Because many of these are consistent with artistic inquiry as well, readers interested in a more thorough examination are referred to Lincoln and Guba's classic *Naturalistic Inquiry* (1985) or Denzin and Lincoln's comprehensive collection, *Handbook of Qualitative Research* (1994). I will however er describe a few basic criteria that are most applicable to an understanding of truth and value within the context of artistic inquiry.

As part of determining truth, the *credibility* and *dependability* (Erlandson, Harris, Skipper, & Allen, 1993) of the source of the data and the methods of gathering it can be assured by a rigorous and thorough description of the methods used. This must include how the participants were selected and the nature of their relationships with the researcher both at the beginning of the study and how the relationships evolved during the inquiry process. It also must assess the *trustworthiness* of the informants. It is recommended that multiple sources of data, forms of data, and persons collecting the data be used, a method called *triangulation* (Berg, 1989), which checks the accuracy of the sources with one another. If possible, researchers may share their data and findings with participants who can confirm its accuracy from their perspective, a process called *member checking* (Erlandson et al., 1993). Consultation with co-researchers, peers, committee members, and advisors throughout the process also assists in verifying that the process did in fact proceed as the researcher describes it. These *peer* and *advisor reviews* can assist the researcher in developing awareness of her or his own biases, which the qualitative paradigm assumes will be active in any research.

Written observations and *reflexive journaling* (Erlandson et al., 1993) during (if appropriate) and after every encounter with the participants and the data, and throughout the data analysis, provides a record of the process and of the evolving understanding of the researcher, who is seen as the primary research tool. The resulting *transparency* of process offers a window into many aspects of the research including the motivations of the researcher(s) and relationships between researchers, participants, and the research context. These notes and all other data records in all forms must be preserved and made available if necessary to provide evidence of the credibility of the research method in the form of an *audit trail* (Erlandson et al., 1993).

Authenticity is probably the qualitative truth criteria most meaningful to dance/movement therapists who wish to do artistic inquiry. It refers to the intentional representation of the realities of all those involved in the design, methods, and presentation of the research (Lincoln & Guba, 1985). The qualitative paradigm is very much concerned with the authentic representation of those traditionally referred to as subjects, who are frequently powerless, anonymous, voiceless and disembodied in the research process and outcomes. I have written elsewhere of my equal concern with researchers, like dance/movement therapists, who are similarly represented inauthentically by forms of research that do not reflect the realities of their practices and experiences (Hervey, 2000).

Dance/movement therapists frequently witness movement as it shifts into something they can identify as authentic. We judge the image, gesture, or sound that rings true, that touches us most profoundly, as authentic. This discernment of authenticity may be the single greatest factor in determining validity of artistic inquiry and yet there is little written that describes exactly *how* it is discerned. Practitioners of authentic movement, an approach to dance/movement therapy, have described it phenomenologically at length (Adler, 1999; Chodorow, 1974/1999; Whitehouse, 1979/1999). Theoretically, there is reason to believe that posture/gesture merger may be an indication of authenticity of movement (Davies, 2001). Much of the recent work of dance/movement therapist Susan Imus has focused on the discernment of authenticity and its relationship to aesthetics (2001). Put simply, she has claimed that authentic *is* aesthetic. Understanding this link may shed light on how intrinsic authenticity is to artistic inquiry. This will be addressed again in the case description of artistic inquiry in this chapter.

The value of any research study to its consumers, and to the field of study to which it attempts to contribute is determined by a number of factors.

Generalizability or *transferability* (Lincoln & Guba, 1985) is a primary concern for artistic inquiry, as it is for any research project. This criterion examines whether the findings of a study with a particular sample can be generalized or transferred to other samples from the same population. Researchers have made a strong case for the idea that qualitative research that is carried out in natural contexts has its own generalizability, arguing that because the events observed were happening naturally, they are very likely to happen again in similar natural contexts. In general, transferability increases as manipulation or control of the research context decreases. Artistic inquiry in natural settings can make similar claims.

More specifically, the question of a study's applicability to clinicians, administrators, or other stakeholders is critical. Unfortunately, because there have been very few artistic inquiries completed in the field of dance/movement therapy to date, the verdict is still very much out on the question and I can only conjecture from those I have witnessed. If an artistic inquiry provides an authentic window into the experiences of therapists and clients, then it would serve to expand the kinesthetic empathy, theoretical understanding, and clinical repertoire of its audience members. This may be a valuable basis upon which to evaluate a work of research. This could also be a particularly valuable method for sharing learning about clients from diverse cultural backgrounds that may be unfamiliar to those witnessing the outcome of the inquiry, as will be illustrated in the thesis described in this chapter.

By definition research is considered valuable when it contributes to the body of knowledge of a field of study. The nature of knowledge in dance/movement therapy is very much grounded in the body (literally), in creativity, and in dance. Perhaps an artistic inquiry can be evaluated by the extent to which it strengthens access to and understanding of these three sources of theory and practice. The results of an artistic inquiry might also be assessed based on the extent to which it reflects the aesthetic values of dance/movement therapy, or evokes what a work of art does: transcendence, meaning, beauty, or joy. Finally, a work of artistic inquiry might be judged by whether it stimulates curiosity and excitement about doing research, a very valuable commodity.

To summarize, the truth and value of an artistic inquiry can be determined by some criteria that have been developed by qualitative researchers, and others that are more unique to art and movement based research methods. The accuracy of the data is confirmed by assuring the credibility of the sources, and by methods such as triangulation and member checking. Thoroughly describing the development and progression of the research methods, using the researchers' notes for details of the process, provides detailed information about the research process and context through transparency. This contributes to the study's transferability, or the likelihood of the described phenomenon occurring among similar samples and in similar contexts. Artistic inquiry offers opportunities for the researcher and the researched to be represented with authenticity, a truth criterion that gives personal truth a high priority.

The remainder of this chapter is a description of an artistic inquiry recently completed by a dance/movement therapy student at Columbia College Chicago. I am deeply grateful to Nancy Toncy for allowing me to witness her research/creative process and consenting to its inclusion here in as much detail as possible. She has agreed that my description is accurate. For a more thorough description of the process and the product, please refer to her master's thesis, which is housed in the Columbia College Chicago Library.

WHAT ARE MUSLIM WOMEN'S EXPERIENCES IN THEIR BODIES IN DANCE/MOVEMENT THERAPY: AN ARTISTIC INQUIRY

Nancy Toncy came to the United States from Cairo, Egypt to study dance/movement therapy at Columbia College Chicago. Before coming to the United States, she was a professional dancer, a dance instructor, and a graduate student of special education. Her dream was to return to Cairo to work as a dance/movement therapist, but she was concerned that the practice of DMT might be so embedded in Western assumptions and ideologies that it would not be acceptable to people in a primarily Muslim culture. One step toward preparing herself for this possibility was to find out how a small sample of women, representing several segments of Muslim culture, experienced a situation like dance/movement therapy. She entered this research with the desire to help women like herself discover greater self-awareness and freedom of self-expression in their worlds (Tonsy, 2003).

As Nancy began her research with a literature review, she quickly became aware of her strong emotional reaction and political position in relation to the literature on the topic of Muslim women and their bodies. Being an Egyptian woman with a Muslim heritage, Nancy's journey to the United States and her training in DMT had already created major shifts in her cultural perceptions about gender role and self-expression through her own body. At these early stages of writing it became clear that her personal experience as a researcher needed to be included as a heuristic component to the research. Heuristic research, as defined by Clark Moustakas (1990), uses the experience of the researcher around a particular event or question as a primary focus and tool of investigation. In this kind of research, the researcher must commit to personal journaling as an essential record of his/her experience, ensuring transparency of process.

While still working on her literature review, she and I (as her research advisor) agreed that artistic inquiry might be the best method for this project, for several reasons. First, because Arabic is Nancy's first language, she does not find her writing in English satisfying or authentic. Second, Nancy's dance technique, choreography skills, aesthetic sense, and commitment to creativity are very strong. Third, it was anticipated that her own and her interviewees' responses to the research question would be rich in emotionally complex, conscious and unconscious material, difficult to translate into quantified or verbal forms. Fourth, because the question was about the experience of the body in context like DMT, much of the data would be nonverbal, visual, and obviously embodied. To remove these data completely from the body, by translating them into narrative description, would sacrifice their essential qualities. Finally, no research on this topic had been conducted before, so there were no findings from which to develop a hypothesis about Muslim women's experiences of or openness to dance/movement therapy.

Data Collection

After completing her review of the literature, Nancy returned to Cairo to gather data. Her sample consisted of twelve women, selected for their diversity of experience within Egyptian Muslim culture, their interest in the research question, and their willingness to participate. None of them was more than an acquaintance of hers.

Nancy initially interviewed each woman, describing her research question at length, and asking for permission to video or audio-tape portions of the interview and movement. Each woman who agreed to participate signed a prepared informed consent statement explaining the nature and purpose of the research, and the extent to which Nancy could ensure confidentiality. Confidentiality was of exceptional importance to these women, who risked their reputations and positions in their communities by revealing themselves physically and sharing their honest feelings. For the women who were normally veiled, the windows of the interview room needed to be covered to insure complete privacy. All interviews were conducted in Arabic to promote authenticity, and were audio-recorded.

The verbal interviews included some or all of the following questions, and others that arose spontaneously from the unstructured dialogue that ensued. The questions assisted Nancy in understanding the context within which each woman lived.

1. What do you spend the most time and energy doing? Your job, being a parent, a homemaker, studying? From which role do you receive the most satisfaction?
2. What are your personal goals?
3. If you could change two aspects of your life, what would you change and how?
4. How did your parents affect or influence the way you have shaped and lived your life so far?

5. How do you fulfill the requirements of your faith (as you interpret them) and live up to religious values in the circumstances and pressures of modern life?
6. What are some of the values and judgments you place onto your body?
7. What are some of the body parts you like/dislike, and why?
8. Why did you choose to wear the hijab? Does wearing the hijab affect you at work or when you commute or within the university?
9. Do veiled and unveiled women have equal opportunities in the society we live in? How does that make you feel?
10. Do you like to dance? What has your dancing experience been like?
11. Where do you actually dance? Does dancing in your private space differ from dancing publicly in social gatherings or weddings?
12. What are some of the important issues or concerns you are currently struggling with?
13. Khuri stated in his book *The Body in Islamic Culture* that "the female body is a source of shame that needs to be covered and concealed." What is your opinion regarding this statement?
14. Were you subjected to any gender inequality or sexual segregation within your family system? How did that make you feel and how did that impact your life in general?
15. How did some of the social restrictions and mandated behaviors imposed by our Arabic culture impact your relational and social development?
16. Is their anything you wish to add? Have I forgotten to ask something that you feel is important? Do you have any questions?

After the verbal interviews, five of the women agreed to participate in one to three movement interview sessions using dance/movement therapy methods. These included a body part and/or body connectivity warm-up; movement into space; gentle encouragement to expand the range of movement; recognition of symbolism and/or memories associated with the movement; and a self-designed closure. Nancy's role was as facilitator and observer, limiting her interventions to reflection, gentle encouragement, clarifications, and open-ended questions about the meanings the women associated with their movement. Because there was no therapeutic contract, the sessions did not have therapeutic goals and did not delve into emotional material, although several of the women did express emotion in response to the interview and the movement experience.

None of the women initially agreed to be videotaped. As a result, Nancy needed a creative solution to preserve their movement as data, to be reviewed and analyzed later. The development of an unprecedented method that met this need is a clear example of the creative process in action in artistic inquiry. Because they had not consented to be videotaped, Nancy realized she had to record herself re-creating the women's move-

ment, as it was the only way she could capture these embodied data for
analysis. She didn't want a third party involved in the sessions, as it might
challenge the women's trust and comfort, especially since confidentiality
was so essential in this context. She also realized that the sooner it could be
done, the more accurate her movement re-creation would be. So, after the
movement interview, Nancy asked each woman to hold the camera and
video-record her for ten minutes as Nancy first explored her own kinesthetic response to the interview, and then for ten minutes attempted to
recall that woman's movements and recreate the dance in her body. The
women were all more than willing to video-record Nancy, and the interactions that arose around the process deepened her relationship with the
women, and led to greater disclosure. It provided an opportunity for the
women to offer her feedback about how accurately she reflected their movements, a form of member checking. Some enjoyed correcting and teasing
her. At least one woman exercised aesthetic choice, zooming in on Nancy
and saying, "Now *I* am making a movie." Evidently this experiment offered
the women a more active role in the research, thereby leading to a greater
sense of empowerment and comfort, and in three cases consent to be videotaped in a second or third movement session was granted.

After watching and recording Nancy's movement responses to their
movements, some of the women asked her questions about why she moved
the way she did. She responded much as a witness in authentic movement
might, taking complete responsibility for her own responses, speaking only
for herself as openly and honestly as she could.

When each movement interview was complete, Nancy wrote detailed
notes about the experience, including all events and her responses to them.
The notes were in English so that they could be used as part of an audit trail
if needed. When Nancy left Cairo she had audio-tapes of all the verbal interviews, video-recordings of herself moving at the end of each of all the movement interviews (recorded by the women), video-recordings of three of the
women moving, and her thorough journal recordings about the entire data
collection process.

Data Analysis

The analysis actually started during the movement interviews, as she
responded to the experience verbally and nonverbally with the women.
Nancy has identified the women as co-researchers because of how active she
felt they were in addressing the research question with her. The experience
of moving with the women, then in response to the women, and finally like
the women, involved kinesthetic empathy, somatic countertransference,
and kinesthetic attunement. These are all frequently used dance/move-
ment therapy methods that can also be considered data analysis methods.
As Nancy observed and moved with the women, she felt kinesthetic empa-

thy in her own body, which gave her information about how the women were feeling as they moved. Similarly, she experienced somatic countertransference, or her own responses that were triggered by the movements, feelings and images expressed by the women. This allowed her to become more conscious of her intrapsychic responses to the unconscious material being presented by the women. When she moved like the women, using kinesthetic attunement and mirroring, both as the women were moving and afterwards as they videotaped her, she began to understand more about the meaning of their movements as well. When she received validation and correction from the women regarding her recreation of their movements, she was checking the accuracy of her data collection and analysis.

After all the interviews were completed, Nancy continued her analysis by talking with advisors and peers, a process that provided ongoing feedback about her personal biases and interpretations. She also wrote and danced about the data and about her experience of the interviews. She noticed that for the weeks following the interviews and again as she worked intensively on creating the dance, she felt "disempowered, unmotivated, tremendously sad, mute—not even present" (personal communication, Feb. 25, 2003). Because these were not her usual affective states, Nancy felt they were somatic countertransference responses to the women's feelings. The data was so rich with unconscious material manifesting in the movement, that she at times felt "foggy," as if she couldn't see or hear. This can be understood as her conscious functioning being overwhelmed by the magnitude of the unconscious material she was processing. It can also be understood as that part of the creative process in which much of the work is done on an unconscious level while the researcher/artist is immersed in intensive conscious effort on the project that may not seem especially effective or productive at the time.

One of the ways Nancy began to work with her countertransference was to dance, finding flamenco a particularly powerful antidote to her disempowering reaction. Its strong, quick rhythms and intense focus may have assisted in reestablishing her boundaries and identity as distinct from the women. During this time she also began her own therapy to assist her in sorting out the conscious and unconscious material that this encounter stimulated, discerning what of it was hers and what belonged to the women she interviewed, and contributing to the authenticity and credibility of the research findings. She continued to journal after every additional dance or encounter with the data that led to new awareness, noting themes that arose in movement, symbol, and word.

I asked Nancy about the relationship between the verbal data from the initial interviews and the movement data. She described the verbal data as representing mostly conscious, cognitive processes that told particular details of each woman's story, such as some of the significant people, events, and conflicts. The movement in contrast was a holistic manifestation, revealing the whole story, in the context of the whole person.

The challenges Nancy faced were a combination of those universally faced by researchers and by artists. Logistically she was challenged around negotiating time and space while enabling her interviewees to attend appointments with her. The more flexible Arabic sense of time impinged upon her need to complete many interviews in a small temporal window. She was also challenged to gather the data in a manner that was respectful of the varied concerns and responses of the interviewees, yet true to her research question. Perhaps the greatest ongoing challenge was discerning her story, her body, her movement, her voice, as distinct from the stories of the women who she interviewed. Finally, she was challenged to create a dance that effectively and accurately represented her own and the women's response to the issues the research question evoked for each of them.

Dance-making

Nancy created a dance that she hoped would reflect the women's responses to the research question asked in so many ways: what is your experience in your body in a context like dance/movement therapy? Her dance-making process involved reviewing the videotapes multiple times, and moving with the women again and again as she watched, until she internalized their unique individual movement styles. She identified and reproduced the most powerful movements and the common themes in the women's movements and symbolic imagery. At one point she said, "They are all different voices, singing the same song." She was challenged to construct a dance that portrayed both the individual women's movement profiles (voices) and their common themes (the song).

I asked Nancy to describe for me, as best she could, *how* she constructed the dance. How did she know when a movement was "right" and should be included in the dance? How did she decide the order in which to put the movements? How did she relate the different women's dances to one another? Her answers were like poetry: passionate, nonlinear, describing an experience embedded in sensory data and intuition.

"When I was with them [the women], I was *so with* them, that my body has the memory." She felt that she *knew* when the movements were right kinesthetically, even without viewing the video recordings, though checking back with the original data was part of ensuring the trustworthiness of the findings. She described her goal as being to find the kinesthetic language of each woman and to make the dance through those languages.

At first, much of the dance-making process seemed to happen in the imaginal realm, where the movements dissolved in and out of Nancy's consciousness, just as the women had moved in and out of her research experience while in Cairo. She tried arranging the movements together purely aesthetically, based on their shape, pace, flow, rhythm, texture. I was reminded of choreographer and dancer Bill T. Jones, who told himself to "just make a beautiful dance, an interesting, vital, challenging dance, and it will say everything that [he] learned," about the people he worked with who had life-threatening diseases (Jones in Moyers, 1997). But Nancy found this method unsatisfactory, empty, void of meaning. She found the "cut and paste" aspects of the method disrespectful of the integrity and wholeness of each woman's story. She found her own aesthetic sense dominating the dance too often.

As the deadline for her performance drew nearer, Nancy began over again, diving back into the data, moving again with the videos of the women. This time she looked for meaningful movement phrases in two ways. First, she examined the ability of the phrase to stand alone in completeness, conveying a whole feeling, story, memory, or image. Secondly, she looked for authenticity of movement. She did not include the abundance of women's movements that seemed like warming up or "getting ready" to move. She began to discriminate between movement that seemed habitual or related to a familiar or defensive social persona, and movement that came from somewhere deeper, more subjective, more personal. It was this latter movement that she was drawn to for its power to communicate something real about the women's experiences of themselves and their relationships to their bodies in the moments she witnessed. At that point in her creative process she was convinced that if she could capture the authenticity of the movements, the aesthetic qualities of the dance would take care of themselves.

Finally, she noticed that when she truly embodied each woman fully, she needed to recuperate from the strangeness of it in her own body. She also needed time to transition from one woman's movement to the next, as it required a dramatic shift from one body ego to the next, neither of which was hers. Thus the dance became a series of vignettes, each a poignant non-verbal message conveyed by unique movement qualities. These were separated by a few moments of deep regulating breath, near stillness, or walking that allowed Nancy to recuperate and prepare for the next woman's movement story. Some of the vignettes were representations of a single woman's very personal story. Others seemed to tell of a universal experience that all of the women shared, and that every audience member could relate to.

The dance evolved into a thirty-minute solo, a long dance by any standards. As beautiful as I found the dance, I knew I was a biased observer, having witnessed the process and Nancy's struggle to transform the data. I was concerned that those in the audience who were not dance/movement therapists might not be as appreciative of the quiet, timeless nature of some of the authentic movement, and might not recognize it as "a dance." I worried it would tax their ability to attend. Nancy had been experimenting with music to use, and had just about given up but I advised that music might help hold the frame of the dance, and hold the aesthetic awareness of the audience. At the time of this writing, Nancy was still looking for the right piece of music to accompany the dance, as she was not happy with the music she chose for the first performance. It needed to be subtle and neutral enough in rhythm so that it would not influence her in the authentic representation of the movement.

Presenting the Findings

The first performance (Hervey & Tonsy, 2003) took place at a professional conference with an audience of Euro-American women, all mental health professionals, many of them dance/movement and creative arts therapists. The room was a medium-sized conference room, with the chairs arranged in proscenium style.

Nancy's stage set consisted of a narrow length of sheer, pale blue fabric hanging vertically from ceiling to floor at an angle to the front of the stage, with which she interacted in symbolic and sensory ways during the dance. Soft, light, flowing, soothing, and sensuous, it became wings, wind, lover, comforter, and *hijab* (veil). She described it as having a spiritual quality at times. Like many props used in dance/movement therapy, the fabric became *the other* in relation to the self in any way that was needed in the performance moment. Subtle music rose and fell intermittently, creating an aura of a very private space. She used her aesthetic values to determine these choices.

Nancy's skills in accurately embodying and re-creating the true qualities of the women's movement made the dance more poignant than a dance performed in a familiar or stylized technique might have been. As a performer, she risked appearing less technically proficient than she actually was as she leaped awkwardly or executed stilted, ungrounded arabesques like those of her co-researchers. The audience responded positively to her dance, describing it in superlatives such as "excellent," "powerful," and "beautiful." Many were struck by the sadness and longing conveyed in the dance.

The dance provided a window through which audience members could gaze at the private experiences of women in another culture. It was left to the viewers to interpret and understand what they saw. A striking paradox became evident between the oppression of Muslim women described in the literature review, the stories of the research participants, and the sensuous, vital beauty of the movement they shared. This is a paradox that Nancy described as pervasive and deeply embedded in her culture. Much of the dialogue before and after the dance performance centered around the differences between Egyptian Muslim and North American women's experiences of oppression, their bodies, and their expressive abilities. Audience members hypothesized about how cultures promote internalized versus externalized oppression. There was also much curiosity about the adaptability of dance/movement therapy to Arabic cultures.

It seemed evident that Nancy's motivating research questions had been answered: Could she be a dance/movement therapist in Cairo? Would Egyptian Muslim women be open to dance/movement therapy? Based on what was discovered in the inquiry, the answers to both questions were yes. It was clear that her co-researchers self-selected to some extent, as only the women who were willing and interested participated in the movement interview. As a result they were probably more open to the movement experience than a random sample of women would have been, challenging the transferability of this study to a wider range of the Muslim women in Egypt. It is reasonable to assume however that a similar self-selection is likely occur when potential clients in Cairo choose dance/movement therapy as their treatment of choice. If dance/movement therapy were offered in an Egyptian psychiatric hospital setting, where patients might not be free to self-select, the response of participants might be strikingly different. However, these same conclusions could be drawn in any culture.

Nancy also came to the realization that adjustments would need to be made to practice dance/movement therapy in a culture that had no established norms defining "appropriate" therapeutic relationships, and a very different awareness than in the United States about the nature of relationships between women in general. Although Cairo was Nancy's home, her understanding of therapy was formed in the United States where basic awareness of the therapeutic relationship and its boundaries are common knowledge. During the interview process Nancy discovered how difficult it was to set culturally sensitive boundaries around time and the extent of her availability to her "co-researchers." In an ongoing therapeutic relationship these boundary issues would very likely be even more challenging. These findings point to the strength of a study done within the cultural context about which there are questions, simulating an experience very close to actual dance/movement therapy with the proposed population.

CONCLUSION

I will close by offering some final conjectures about the value of this example of artistic inquiry in particular and the viability of the research method in general. First and foremost, the commitment and courage required by this work cannot be overstated. There was no way I could have prepared Nancy for the demands of the inquiry process. It could not have succeeded with any less stamina, skill, creativity, and intensity. This is not a method for those who are looking for an easy or fun way out of long, arduous work.

The power of Nancy's dance was undeniable, due primarily I believe to the quality of her performance, her devotion to the creative process, her commitment to the authenticity of the women's dances, and the compelling nature of her research question. The performance was accompanied by a written description of the research questions and method, and discussion before and after the performance, both of which contributed to the effectiveness of its message. I was reminded of how people love to talk about art, theater, dance, et cetera. Good art stimulates lively conversation, rich with analyses and hypotheses. Nancy's dance clearly did that as well. Perhaps evocation of wonder, insight, curiosity, debate, and creativity is one of the functions of artistic inquiry.

Obviously there are challenges to doing this kind of inquiry, as there are in all research methods. The demands on the time, energy, and creativity of the researcher have been stated. The effectiveness of its communication and the utility of its outcomes to audiences must be evaluated case by case. The value of the *method* may in fact need to be considered separately from the value of the *findings*, as they may provide different functions for the profession. Artistic inquiry in all its myriad forms, may prove to be a challenging, motivating, and growthful process for those who engage in, contribute to, and witness it. The outcomes of the best inquiries may prove as puzzling and awesome as art itself, with all the same rewards. More opportunities are needed to have dialogues with creators and consumers of this research about what is being conveyed and how. If I may return to my opening birth metaphor, artistic inquiry is just being born into our field. Its viability and stability are yet to be determined. We are witnessing its first breaths, and have much to learn.

REFERENCES

Adler, J. (1999). Integrity of body and psyche. In P. Pallaro (Ed.). *Authentic movement.* (pp. 121–131). Philadephia, PA: Jessica Kingsley.

Barone, T., & Eisner, E. (1997). Arts-based educational research. In R. Jaeger (Ed.) *Complementary methods for research in education.* (pp. 73–116). Washington, DC: American Educational Research Association.

Berg, B. B. (1989). *Qualitative research methods.* Boston, MA: Allyn &Bacon.

Braud, W., & Anderson, R. (1998). *Transpersonal research methods for the social sciences.* Thousand Oaks, CA: Sage.

Bronson, P. (2002). *What should I do with my life?* New York: Random House.

Chodorow, J. (1974/1999). Philosophy and methods in individual work. In P. Pallaro(Ed.), *Authentic movement* (pp. 229–235). Philadelphia, PA: Jessica Kingsley.

Davies, E. (2001). *Beyond dance: Laban's legacy of movement analysis.* London: Brechen Books.

Denzin, N. K., & Lincoln, Y. S. (1994). *Handbook of qualitative research.* Thousand Oaks, CA: Sage.

Eisner, E. (1991). *The enlightened eye.* New York: Macmillan.

Eisner, E. (1995). What artistically crafted research can help us understand about schools. *Educational Theory, 45*(1), 1–6.

Eisner, E. (1997). The new frontier in qualitative research methods. *Qualitative Inquiry, 3*(3), 259–273.

Erlandson, D. A., Harris, E. L., Skipper, B. L., & Allen, S. D. (1993). *Doing naturalistic inquiry: A guide to methods.* Newbury Park, CA: Sage.

Feynman, R. (1985/1997). The dignified professor. In F. Barron, A. Montuori, & A. Barron (Eds.), *Creators on creating* (pp. 63–67). New York: Putnam Sons.

Gadamer, H. G. (1998). *Truth and method,* (2nd ed. rev.). New York: Continuum.

Hervey, L. (2000). *Artistic inquiry in dance/movement therapy: Creative research alternatives.* Springfield, IL: Charles C Thomas.

Hervey, L., & Tonsy, N. (2003). Muslim women's experiences in their bodies: An artistic inquiry through dance/movement therapy. Presented at the Midwest Expressive Arts Therapy Festival. Lake Geneva, WI.

Imus, S. (2001). Aesthetics and authentic: The art in dance/movement therapy. *Proceedings after the 36th Annual Conference of the American Dance Therapy Association,* Raleigh, NC. Columbia, MD: American Dance Therapy Association.

Janesick, V. J. (1994). The dance of qualitative research design. In N. K. Denzin & Y. S. Lincoln (Eds.), *Handbook of qualitative research.* (pp. 209–219). Thousand Oaks, CA: Sage.

Jimenez-Figueroa, I. (2003). *Danzando en Espanol: Moving in Spanish. Dance/movement therapy with Hispanic/Latino immigrants dealing with acculturation.* Unpublished proposal. Columbia College Chicago.

Lewis, P. (1984). *Theoretical approaches in dance/movement therapy.* Dubuque, IA: Kendall/Hunt.

Lincoln, Y., & Guba, E. (1985). *Naturalistic inquiry.* Thousand Oaks, CA: Sage.

McNiff, S. (1987). Research and scholarship in the creative arts therapies. *The Arts in Psychotherapy, 14*(2), 285–292.

McNiff, S. (1993). The authority of experience. *The Arts in Psychotherapy, 20,* 3–9.

McNiff, S. (1998). *Art-based research.* London: Jessica Kingsley.

Moustakas, C. (1990). *Heuristic research.* Newbury Park, CA: Sage.

Moyers, B. (1997). *Bill T. Jones: Still /Here with Bill Moyers.* Princeton, NJ: Films of the Humanities and Sciences.

Nachmanovitch, S. (1990). *Free play.* New York: G.P. Putnam's Sons.

Oldfather, P., & West, J. (1994). Qualitative research as jazz. *Educational Researcher, 23*(8), 22–26.

Poincare, H. (1908/1952). Mathematical creation. In B. Ghiselin (Ed.). *The Creative Process* (p. 33). New York: New American Library.

Reason, P., & Rowan, J. (Eds.) (1981). *Human inquiry.* Chichester, UK: John Wiley.

Shekerjian, D. (1990). *Uncommon genius: Tracing the creative impulse with forty winners of the MacArthur Award.* New York: Viking.

Stinson, S. (1995). Body of knowledge. *Educational Theory, 45*(1): 43–54.

Strauss, A., & Corbin, J. (1990*). Basics of qualitative research: Grounded theory procedures and techniques.* Thousand Oaks, CA: Sage.

Tonsy, N. (2003). *The voices of Muslim women as heard through their bodies.* Unpublished proposal. Columbia College Chicago.

Wallas, G. (1926). *The art of thought.* New York: Harcourt-Brace. *Webster's New Collegiate Dictionary.* (1981). Springfield, MA: G. & C. Merriam Company.

Whitehouse, M. (1979/1999). C.G. Jung and dance therapy: Two major principles. In P. Pallaro (Ed.). *Authentic movement.* (pp. 73–101). Philadelphia, PA: Jessica Kingsley.

Chapter 12

HOW TO MIX QUANTITATIVE
AND QUALITATIVE METHODS IN A DANCE/
MOVEMENT THERAPY RESEARCH PROJECT

Cynthia F. Berrol

INTRODUCTION

No matter the paradigm or specific model employed, the most abiding aspect of research is that it is simply the act of seeking and acquiring knowledge through exploration and discovery. One has only to look at a salient exemplar, child development, to witness the inherent genesis of problem solving and to understand how mixed methods nourish, sustain and advance its unfolding. An underlying question is what kindles the innate and enduring desire to question, search, and discover.

Stewart (1987, 2001) and Chodorow (1991, in press) offer that the two positive innate affects, interest and joy, are dynamically expressed through curiosity and play, respectively. Through their corollary ego functions, exploration and fantasy (creative imagination), humans are primed for what we label research.

Progressing a step further, it is possible to synthesize Piaget's theory of cognitive development (Piaget & Inhelder, 1969), starting with the sensorimotor stage, (ages 0-2 years), and Stewart's theory of the development of ego function (2001). This period of extraordinary and rapid early child development advances from purely reflexive reactions to purposeful behaviors. Beginning with trial and error exploration, the preverbal infant/toddler begins to discover and understand his or her world, primarily through movement activity. Stewart speaks of this process as the dynamic interplay between two innate affects, "interest-curiosity/exploration and joy-play/fantasy" (p. 70), the driving forces of cognitive and symbolic development.

It is possible to conceive of the child as an imaginative inquirer, exploring and problem solving within the parameters of his or her environment, drawing upon the inherent affects of curiosity and interest (Chodorow, in press; Stewart, 2001). The process may start inductively (imputing meaning from trial and error discoveries), taking form and shape as discoveries are made and patterns of behavior/action emerge—what Piaget terms "schema"—and what can loosely be equated with formulations of theory. In children the inquiry process is an ongoing dance between inductive and deductive methods. The latter builds on already learned patterns, somewhat akin to a prediction; that is, if I do *this* then it will probably make *that* happen, a cause–effect relationship. Beginning at a rudimentary, concrete level, with advancing age the level of cognition progresses to abstract thinking and hypothesizing—the mature stage of cognitive development or formal operations (Piaget & Inhelder, 1969). This intrinsic learning mechanism seems a microcosm of what formal research inquiry is all about—the interplay between inductive and deductive paradigms, reflections on emergent questions, and the various and most feasible strategies for seeking answers. With this model in mind, I transition to mixing research methods as a viable option in a study.

Research inquiry exists in many guises, from predictive, objective, and measurable forms to interpretive, contextual, and subjective modes. Much has been written in recent years about the diverse options open to the creative arts therapies relative to scholarly investigation (Edwards, 1999; McNiff, 1998; Gantt, 1998; Spaniol, 1998; Julliard, 1998; Bloomgarten, 1998; Forinash, 1995; Junge & Linesch, 1993; Hervey, 2000). Perhaps past issues surrounding the historically cool relationship between dance/movement therapy (DMT) and research may be linked to the lack of a clear understanding of the vast spectrum of credible inquiry alternatives that are available. I refer here to techniques that extend beyond the parameters of experimentally designed studies, specifically to qualitative (also known as phenomenologic or interpretive) approaches. The point of emphasis here, regardless of the model or paradigm favored, is enriching the body of knowledge through creative problem solving and discovery (i.e., credible investigative research is the overarching goal of most disciplines and certainly of DMT).

Similarly, current articles and books have probed the nature of research inquiry in dance and the creative arts therapies with respect to underlying philosophical, theoretical, and methodological tenets and practices (Lincoln & Guba, 1985; Cook & Reichardt, 1979; McNiff, 1998; Junge & Linesch, 1993; Politsky, 1995; Hanstein, 1999; Hervey, 2000). In this chapter, quantitative and qualitative inquiry, two differing philosophical and methodological research frameworks, are highlighted within the context of their respective overarching paradigms—deductive and inductive logic. These vehicles for research are compared and incorporated into a spectrum of possible combinations for use in DMT research inquiry.

The approach of mixing research methods has recently gained attention in the annals of research literature (Tashakkori & Teddlie, 1998; Neuman & Benz, 1998; Walizer & Wienir, 1978; Cresswell, 1994). Simply, this refers to the combining of approaches and paradigms within the same study or during different phases of the same study.

The various proponents of mixed methods emphasize that the type of research questions posed ultimately determines the mode of inquiry warranted and unveils different perspectives of the same issue—a kaleidoscopic revelation of sorts. Within this context, the issue of matching objectives with appropriate methodological approaches is addressed and illuminated by practical examples of studies in which authors have incorporated mixed methods into their research designs. Although some of the various research options applied in quantitative and qualitative inquiries are touched upon here, they will not be fully amplified as other chapters probe these different approaches.

RESEARCH DEFINED

Webster's New World Dictionary (Guralnik, 1992) defines research as careful and critical inquiry and examination for the purpose of discovery and interpretation of new knowledge to increase our understanding of the world. In essence, it is a pursuit that has preoccupied humankind since the beginning of recorded time.

More specifically, Junge and Linesch (1993) conceive of research as "structured inquiry" employing appropriate methods "for the purpose of producing reliable and valid knowledge" (p. 63). While this places greater emphasis on form, structure, and methods than the first definition, the commonality is the quest to unravel and comprehend the mysteries of the human experience.

OVERVIEW OF RESEARCH APPROACHES

Scientific and phenomenological inquiry, the primary research models in the behavioral and social sciences, can be viewed as counterparts. The scientific approach is most associated with quantitative formats and embraces measurable, observable phenomena related to the human experience; qualitative methods look inward at the process of experiencing. One seeks to explain and predict behavior, the other to understand and to interpret it. Together these seemingly polar vehicles can converge to form an holistic portrait of human behavior. Simply, both are needed for a comprehensive view of DMT in terms of what it is, what it does or can do, and in particular, how it works.

In addition, it is important to understand that overlaying the inherent nature and process of the two inquiry methods are two distinct paradigms of reasoning. Quantitative approaches are shaped by deductive logic, and qualitative by inductive logic (Neuman & Benz, 1998). Both evolve from the same starting point—questions seeking resolution. After the initial questions are crystallized, the ensuing steps may, to greater or lesser degrees, begin to diverge.

The term positivism is often associated with quantitative research, and the term postpositivism with qualitative research. The latter moniker was adopted to indicate that it postdated positivism chronologically not because it was similar philosophically (Reichardt & Rallis, 1994). However, current literature indicates that this term is already outmoded, superseded by others denoting specific perspectives such as "constructivist research" (Hedrick, 1994; also see Green in this volume). For the sake of clarity, in this chapter, the labels quantitative and qualitative will be used, primarily, to distinguish the two modes of research with regard to use of theoretical constructs, philosophical concepts, method, data collection, and analysis. I will also differentiate the two research models according to the overarching paradigms generally associated with them, that is, deductive logic with quantitative inquiry and inductive logic with qualitative inquiry. I begin with a brief review of each approach.

Quantitative Research: Experimental and Quasi-experimental Methods

The chapter on quantitative research in this text (Chapter 3, Berrol) described experimental and quasi-experimental approaches as forms of the scientific method. Characterized as a systematic, linear approach that resides in the realm of deductive logic, this type of reasoning begins with a research question that frequently poses an hypothetical question involving cause-effect relationships derived from an established set of related concepts. Adhering to carefully structured procedures, the inquiry sets out to verify (or refute) a theoretically derived prediction (Kerlinger, 1973). The research is designed to test hypotheses by way of a step-by-step progression under regulated conditions. It's characterized as an objective mode in which the researcher formulates research questions and selects related variables; directs and scrutinizes the process; collects and analyzes the data; and finally, discusses and interprets the results. A particular phenomenon is manipulated in a way(s) to trigger a particular effect. The ultimate goal— by way of ongoing investigative replication—is to reveal knowledge in the form of a fact or facts. In the field of medicine, for example, scientists are constantly searching to identify the underlying causes of specific conditions and in the process, to rule out potential competing, but unconfirmed theoretical explanations. In order to confirm the validity of a prediction and to generalize its results, ongoing replications of the research are needed.

This mode of research strives to amplify existing theoretical constructs or to generate new ones. The role of the researcher is that of a witness to the action rather than a participant in it. As pointed out in Chapter 3 of the text, one of the hallmarks of experimental research is quantification of the variables being researched so that statistical tests may be conducted to determine whether or not a predicted relationship can be supported. Even an hypothesis that has survived many replications may still be replaced by newer findings or have alternate, acceptable possibilities.

Whereas pure experimental design adheres to the tightly controlled protocols of laboratory science, quasi-experimental research may be viewed as a more pliable version of this model. Associated with the human sciences, it takes place outside the realm of the laboratory setting so that real life issues can be studied in the context in which they occur. For example, responses to psychosocial treatments such as psychotherapy should take place in the hospitals and clinics in which these services are provided. The difficulty lies in teasing out and controlling for different internal and external conditions that may affect, obscure, or otherwise skew the outcomes of the research (Borg & Gall, 1979; Borg, Gall, & Gall, 1993). Thus in quasi-experimental approaches, various adjustments and arguments must be logically constructed to rule out competing hypotheses purported to explain the research findings. Efforts must be made to accommodate the multilayered realities of exploring the domains of human behavior and function while establishing a rationale for the validity of the research. However, most researchers agree that there is no ultimate proof of a research outcome.

Qualitative Research

Alternatively known as phenomenological or interpretive research, this method has been propelled by recognition that the laws governing the natural sciences may not always be applicable to the behavioral and social sciences. Qualitative research embraces the notion that knowledge is fallible, a human creation, and that the intricate web of dynamics impacting critical dimensions of human behavior may elude linear quantification. Rather than accepting assumptions of linear causality, qualitative inquiry embraces the notion of a world view predicated on "mutual causality" or "multiple realities," one in which ongoing dynamic relationships among phenomena preclude linear modes of quantification (Lincoln & Guba, 1985; Moustakas, 1994; Edwards, 1999).

This method, with roots in the ancient world, is related to "hermeneutics," a form of inquiry derived from Hermes, the messenger of the Greek gods who communicated the gods' messages to mortals (Neuman & Benz, 1998). Historically, hermeneutics is portrayed as an approach concerned with unraveling and making meaning of esoteric texts (philosophic, historic, or religious).

In qualitative research the emphasis is on studying people in real life situations. The researcher strives to probe the substance and meaning of the human experience, to gain insights into the perceptions of individuals, groups, cultures and organizations. This research model attempts to stretch the limitations of quantitative methods. Process oriented, the researcher reflects the perspective of the one who is experiencing and, importantly, interprets and imputes meaning to those experiences, events, and activities under study (Edwards, 1999; Berrol, Ooi, & Katz, 1997; Moustakas, 1994; Junge & Linesch, 1993).

Two Overarching Paradigms: Deductive and Inductive Logic

Whereas the scientific model is tied to deductive reasoning, qualitative design is grounded in inductive reasoning. One of the defining differences between the two is that a deductive approach is concerned with witnessing and reporting on what is happening —i.e., the product—whereas an inductive approach concentrates on understanding and interpreting the underlying process. According to Moustakas (1994), an inductive paradigm is generally not predicated on a priori assumptions or pre-selected variables but rather resides with the researcher who formulates a guiding question or problem—i.e., the "phenomenon." Inductive logic extracts and distills ideas or premises embedded in the collected narratives of descriptive field data for objectification and interpretation. This approach may be compared to a sculptor whose creation emerges from the raw material rather than something he or she imposes upon it. This image is congruent with the distinction dancers and dance/movement therapists make between "I move" and "I am moved"—the sense of being propelled by an internal catalyst.

A qualitative format revolves around gathering descriptive narrative from the participants of the study (sometimes referred to as "co-researchers"), and documenting and using an assortment of data collection tools (e.g., formal or informal interviews, surveys and field observations, film and video). The collected information is then readied for scrupulous analysis for unifying themes, patterns and importantly, meaning, and ultimately configured to induce theories or hypotheses reflective of the particular participants studied (Moustakas, 1994; Lincoln & Guba, 1985). These studies, considered "context bound," are rooted in "grounded theory," implying that the propositions educed are extracted from within the context of the natural field and modified as other data emerge to reshape the "concepts, focus or direction of the questions" (Neuman & Benz, 1998, p. 146).

Methods vary, depending on the phenomena being examined and the underlying objectives of the investigator. Green and Horton (1999) observe that not all post-positivists share congruent perspectives; basic assumptions or methodological procedures, and even the role of the researcher may differ. Among the modes of qualitative research now in evidence are: action, feminist, heuristic, ethnologic, hermeneutic, anthropologic, and participatory. The fluid nature of this paradigm reflects a still evolving state, contouring to fit the conditions and nature of the inquiry along with the philosophic stance of the researcher.

Regardless of the diverse forms of data gathering, the *investigator* is the instrument of, as well as the interpreter of, the results. Meaning is ultimately shaped by two interacting factors, the raw descriptive data reflecting the perceptions of the participants, and the analytic interpretations constructed through the lens of the investigator. Forinash (1995) depicts qualitative research as relational; the researcher is not detached from the phenomena and carries his or her personal perspective to the research event. The researcher, rather than an objective eyewitness, is as an active presence, one of the change agents in the psycho-social dynamics of the phenomena under study (Junge & Linesch, 1993).

Dance anthropologist Judith Hanna comments (in Chapter 9 of this text) on the difficulty ethnological researchers have maintaining neutral and objective in field research as they probe for "facts and truths." She contends that they must be aware of and acknowledge personal biases, motives, and behaviors that may impact the research process. This may be akin to the dance/movement therapist identifying and dealing with transference and counter transference issues that arise in the therapeutic interaction.

A striking example of researcher bias as depicted by Ekman (1998) concerns famed anthropologist Margaret Mead and her stance on human nature and the environment. In synchrony with an era that embraced nurture over nature, Ekman informs that Mead concluded, "human nature was almost unbelievably malleable," (p. 168) and that the impact of the cultural environment was limitless. Biology was ignored as an influencing factor. Ekman maintains that Mead's one-sided view was based on a conscious decision she had made "not to consider the biological aspect of behavior because of the political problems it would cause" (p. 168).

Thus, in an approach vulnerable to researcher bias, protocols for interpretative analysis need be quite rigorous to maintain the integrity and credibility of an inquiry—the counterpart of validity in scientific research. An excellent example of meticulous attention to accuracy in qualitative research may be found in Rehavia-Hanauer's (2003) art therapy study in which conflicts of individuals with anorexia nervosa are identified through the art therapy process. She describes the different stages of fleshing-out, analyzing and interpreting the raw data for recurrent themes, categorizing, re-categorizing, and synthesizing the data into meaningful units. The final stage of the research details the scrupulous evaluation procedures used to obtain the results to insure validity. In addition, Forinash's chapter on qualitative methods in this text provides a comprehensive chronicling of a content analysis and validation procedures of a DMT research study with frail elderly individuals.

Table 12-I offers a comparative summary of quantitative and qualitative methods.

MIXING RESEARCH METHODS

With the basic premises and distinctions between the two primary research paradigms recapped, the notion of mixing research methods is now explored with respect to what it is, and why and how it is used.

Table 12-I   COMPARISON OF QUANTITATIVE AND QUALITATIVE RESEARCH

Categories	Quantitative Research	Qualitative Research
Goals of researcher	Facts, truths, and explanations related to natural and behavioral sciences	Meaning, understanding, and interpretation of the data
Paradigm	Deductive reasoning based on established theoretical constructs	Inductive reasoning based on gathering data to formulate theoretical constructs
Type of data collected	Typically quantifiable: outcome oriented, verifiable, reliable	Process oriented: descriptive, narrative
Type of data analysis	Statistical analyses: comparisons of two or more groups on selected variables; often involves causal relationships	Descriptive analyses: field observations, formal and informal interviews, videos, photos, film
Characteristics of researcher	Researcher removed from data; works from without—objective, noninteractive observer	Researcher close to data, works from within—interactive observer/participant
Characteristics of research	Objective, value free, rational, accurate, valid, reliable, factual	Personal, based on participants' subjective experiences and perceptions; verifiable
Attributes of research model	Deductive logic—reductionist: tries to rule out or eliminate alternative causal theories; hypothesis testing; interpretative based on data finding, making inferences	Inductive logic—expansionist: descriptive, interpretative, finding meaning
Nature of research	Generalizable with adequate replication studies: predictions and inferences; amplification and/or formulations of theory	May be "transferable" but not generalizable: propositions formulated from patterns and themes; time and context bound—small samples; site specific

Note: Ideas for Table 12-I were adapted from Cook & Reinhardt (1979, p. 10); and Politsky, (1995, pp. 308). The quantitative portion of the table is extrapolated from Chapter 3, Table 1 (Basic Characteristics of Quantitative Research) and juxtaposed here to visually illuminate and examine core differences between the two paradigms.

What Is It?

Tashakkori and Teddlie (1998) characterize mixed methods as a pragmatic model with no set concepts about truth or reality. The authors perceive it as a form that combines different inquiry methods within a research investigation to adequately address a question or different questions that call for quantitative as well as qualitative data gathering and analysis. Various authors cited in this chapter comment that advances in computer hardware and software programs have helped to boost the use of mixed models. Computer programs are available for quantitative analysis of statistical data as well as for content analysis of interpretative data.

Why Is It Used?

First, consideration needs to be given to the inherent nature of each research model and its potential for meeting the demands of the inquiry, that is, its intent and the nature of the emergent questions. We have already established that quantitative designs examine what happens when a particular phenomenon is acted upon by measuring the observable effects, and that qualitative modes focus on why, exploring and explaining the underlying processes shaping the events. The two functions are not independent of each other but rather address different perspectives or questions regarding the same phenomena (Tashakkori & Teddlie, 1998). Each method serves to amplify and inform the other in a complementary union.

How Is It Used?

Basic to the application of mixed methods is the concept of "triangulation," which simply means the use of more than one method to collect and analyze data on the same variables or phenomena (Neuman & Benz, 1998; Cresswell, 1994; Tashakkori & Teddlie, 1998). According to Cresswell (1994), combining methods in a single study was originally conceived to neutralize investigator bias. This mix offered a malleable model that could be manipulated in various ways, depending on the emergent questions and purposes. Creswell (1994) informs that the initial rationale for triangulation has broadened from controlling research bias to deepening and enriching the scope and depth of the research, an effect he terms "expansion" (p. 175). He observes that the combination of designs offers "complementary" facets of the same variables; augments the inquiry "developmentally" with one phase of the research informing the next; and acts as a catalyst for "initiation" or opportunities for "contradictions, paradoxes and fresh perspectives to emerge" (p. 175).

Possibilities for mixing different research designs vary with the project. There are instances during the process of an inquiry when a researcher discovers that an additional but related method would be important to integrate into the research. Likewise, mixing different paradigms in the same investigation is an option in the mixed methods container (see Samples 3 and 4 below). A researcher might combine two different stages of a research project such as a study of the effect of a treatment like DMT (framed by deductive logic) with in-depth interviews (tethered to an inductive paradigm). Tashakkori and Teddlie (1998) state that during the different stages of the research process, qualitative data may be converted to quantitative and vice versa. Survey data within a single study may include closed-ended objective questions (quantitative) as well as open-ended narrative—qualitative—inquiries (see Sample 2 below).

The sequence, type, and number of combinations possible for mixing methods depend on the overarching design of the study and are organized according to the unfolding demands of the research. Data gathered in one phase may indicate the need for another type of analysis or approach in another phase. This multifaceted form is configured to meet the emergent exigencies of the research project. Since there is no single template for combining paradigms and methods, several samples will be presented to illustrate how various researchers have—without labeling them as such— incorporated aspects of mixed methods into their studies.

Research Samplings

Sample 1

An art therapy case study of adolescent girls with anorexia nervosa was conducted in a hospital employing qualitative data collection and analytic procedures within a deductive paradigm. Art therapist Rehavia-Hanauer (2003) explored and identified underlying causes of conflicts associated with anorexia nervosa as they were reflected in ten adolescent females through the art therapy process. After a background introduction that established the purpose of her study, the researcher presented a thorough and well documented review of literature that spanned a comprehensive spectrum of theoretical models dealing with the genesis of anorexia.

The role of the literature review in this study clearly establishes a deductive paradigm. To amplify the deductive rationale, the review of literature comes early on in the research process (see the Literature Review section of Chapter 3 in this text). It identifies and presents established theories to construct a rationale for the study and to support concepts directly related to the research topic. Although a review of literature is a standard component of all inquiries, in inductive paradigms, when and how it is integrated into the study is dependent upon the global design of the research.

Based on this distinction, Rehavia-Hanauer's (2003) review of literature adopted the structure of a deductive paradigm. However, data collection and analysis clearly fall into the domain of a qualitative analysis. Detailed narrative data, collected over an extended period of time, were content analyzed to flesh-out basic conflicts linked with anorexia nervosa. Moreover, the author chronicled the process of verifying the interpretation of the content analysis enlisting one of the methods associated with establishing the credibility of a qualitative inquiry. These procedures are characteristic of an inductive paradigm.

Finally, the researcher returned to the deductive paradigm by directly linking each of the identified conflictual issues to one or more of the psychoanalytic theories highlighted in the review of literature and interpreting them within that context. The importance of connecting the outcome of the research to its theoretical underpinnings is one of the hallmarks of a deductive paradigm.

Augmenting the potential variants of mixed methods, some investigations might reflect a fairly even division between the different modes, while in other instances one or another may predominate. The study summarized above clearly resembles the latter in that it is qualitative in intent and for the most part in procedure—specifically, clinical procedures, data collection, and data analytic methods. In addition, the means of establishing the integrity of the data analysis embraced a qualitative model. Nevertheless, the literature review, which established the theoretical constructs of the inquiry, and relationship of the content analysis to the theoretical premises were grounded in a deductive paradigm. Although qualitative in terms of the method, when carefully scrutinized, the study falls into the category of mixed methods research—i.e., a qualitative design housed in a deductive paradigm.

Sample 2

A survey of members of the American Dance Therapy Association (Cruz & Hervey, 2001) was conducted regarding therapists' attitudes toward research and their perceptions of the importance of research in clinical practice. The study combines quantitative[1] and qualitative methods.

Cruz and Hervey divided the survey into two parts: quantitative and qualitative, respectively. The first part of the questionnaire comprised several categories, beginning with multiple response items, age of therapist, and clinical populations served. A series of yes/no questions addressed clinical work settings, research training, research involvement, computer/electronic mail experience, and professional practice items. Several questions regarding perceived barriers to "carrying out research" were divided into "Not a Barrier," "Small Barrier," "Significant Barrier," and "Large Barrier" (p. 99). The data from the objective portion of the survey were calculated as frequencies to establish how responses to the various questions were distributed among the sample group and then reported as percentages.

The second portion of the survey, designed for narrative responses, requested that respondents who had been involved in a research project and/or had applied for a grant describe certain aspects of the process. These overlapped with the objective (yes/no) questions that addressed specific facets of the respondents' experiences with research, for example, if the individual had ever engaged in a research project, had collaborated on one, had worked independently on one, had designed one, et cetera. Some final open-ended questions invited respondents to express attitudes and feelings concerning research and likewise, to share their perceptions of its value to their practices as well as to the profession. The qualitative data were content analyzed to extract and synthesize core points that emerged.

When juxtaposed, the findings of the objective portion revealed the frequency of occurrences of specific research-related issues, and the subjective part amplified parallel aspects of them. These open-ended questions unmasked a somewhat equivocal finding: while respondents felt that

---

[1]The quantitative aspects of the survey were examined in Chapter 3.

research had little practical value in their own clinical work they perceived research as very important to the profession.

The study represents mixed methods within survey research in which the quantitative and qualitative components played complementary roles. Although the objective questions significantly outnumbered the qualitative, the latter were far more time consuming to answer and provided important subjective insights about the respondents' thoughts, attitudes, and feelings regarding the research issue.

Sample 3

A research study examining the effects of DMT with older individuals who had sustained neurotrauma (traumatic brain injury and stroke) (Berrol, Ooi, & Katz, 1997) presents yet another example of the use of mixed methods. The investigation was conducted in ten different facilities—from residential to day treatment centers—across five different geographic regions.

Grounded in a deductive paradigm, the general design of the investigation was representative of quantitative research—specifically quasi-experimental—in addition to a quantitative survey. Related qualitative dimensions were incorporated to amplify the implications of the statistical findings. Although no formal hypotheses were formulated, the underlying assumption was that DMT would assist in the amelioration of a number of key problems associated with insult to the brain.

The quantitative variables examined were selected measures of physical function, cognitive status, mood, and social interaction. Pre and posttest measures were statistically analyzed to discern differences within and between the two sample groups that could be attributed to the experimental condition.

A survey, described as a posttreatment patient satisfaction questionnaire, was developed to assess the experimental group's satisfaction with the intervention and their perceptions of its effect on their social interactions and functional abilities. Primarily a "yes/no/don't know" format, the responses were tabulated and reported as percentages.

Qualitative data were gathered from two sources: a) ten summative reports, written in narrative form (including anecdotal data), submitted by the eight dance/movement therapists hired to conduct the intervention; and b) analyses of three videotaped sessions of two groups from the California sites. Therapists' evaluations of the therapeutic process vis-à-vis targeted intervention variables were content analyzed for common themes and underscored as significant factors associated with the DMT intervention.

According to Berrol, Ooi, and Katz (1997), findings from all the data sources were reviewed for congruencies in relation to the targeted intervention variables: physical and cognitive function; mood/depression; social interaction; and active participation. For example, therapists documented increased physical ambulation of the subjects and for "progressively longer periods." Concurrently, the quantitative analysis registered statistically meaningful change on several walking measures favoring the experimental group over the controls. Similarly the patient survey revealed that a significant proportion of the participants felt better physically—in balance, leg strength, and reduction of physical pain. This was supplemented by anecdotal accounts documented in the therapists' final reports. "I always feel better after dancing, even if I'm not feeling so good when I come," "This will hold me over till next time" (p. 159). During check-in at the start of one session, a patient commented, "I feel like a cloudy day with a lightning bolt through it." At closing she shared, "I feel perky now" (p. 158).

In another instance of data concordance, dance/movement therapists commented on improvements observed in patients' memories during movement sequencing activities, noting as well an increasing use of imagery during sessions. These observations correlated with significant quantitative differences detected on the cognitive scale, favoring the experimental group over the controls.

The dependent variable, social interaction, revealed significant quantitative improvement for the experimental group. This statistical finding was congruent with the therapists' accounts of increased bonding over time in terms of friendships; sharing and exchanging of memories and feelings; talking about family and problems; and inquiring about absent members. Corollary to these reports and the types of behaviors measured in the social interaction scale, the researchers observed that the videos captured striking examples of how individuals supported and encouraged each other. "Come on, you can do it. I couldn't walk after my stroke and look at me now. You can do it too," "Look how much better you're walking" (Berrol, Katz, & Ooi, pp. 159–160). These observations were similarly supported by the number of positive responses to questions in the survey that focused on friendship, and interaction with others.

The mix of data analyses facilitated a cross-validation of the outcomes that served to support and strengthen the power of the respective findings. Second, and of substantial import, the incorporation of qualitative dimensions furnished insights that more fully illuminated the unfolding therapeutic process and rendered multilayered findings. The various quantitative measures generated hard outcome data representing key aspects of function related to neurotrauma, while the qualitative dimensions furnished an increased understanding of the unfolding therapeutic process as perceived by the therapists and the participants.

Sample 4

A research inquiry examining the use of authentic movement on women's psychological adaptation to breast cancer involved a total of thirty-three women and was conducted in two different geographic locations in the Bay Area of California.

Similar to the previous example, this experimental design (Dibbell-Hope, 2000) followed a standard deductive paradigm. Dibbell-Hope posed research questions, reviewed relevant literature, and unlike the study in Sample 3, she stated directional hypotheses—the main one predicting that women in the authentic movement group would evidence greater improvement than those in the control group (those waiting for treatment). Objective and subjective measures were employed. Quantitative indices comprised four different self report questionnaires evaluating, respectively: affective states; distress states; self concept/body-image; and tendency to over inflate one's social desirability to others.

Qualitative measures were based on in-depth pre- and post-treatment interviews. The first interview contained demographic questions to prepare a profile of the person and questions related to participants' experiences with cancer and feelings regarding their body image. The post treatment interview consisted of two parts, a semi-structured interview and a written evaluation designed for feedback about each person's experiences with the intervention and "how it had affected her feelings about her body and herself," (Dibbell-Hope, 2000, p. 56).

The pre- and posttests of the quantitative data were statistically analyzed to determine whether the treatment outcomes supported the predicted hypotheses. The collated narratives underwent different stages of content analysis, first extracting themes in common, then grouping them on the basis of negative or positive tenor, and finally sequencing the themes by the frequency of occurrence.

In this study, the researcher found distinctive discrepancies between the quantitative and qualitative outcomes. Dibbell-Hope (2000) reported that while the objective data revealed a few changes in mood and distress, no positive changes were discerned on body image or self esteem measures favoring the experimental group. On the other hand, the content analysis of the oral interviews and written evaluations indicated the women perceived noticeable improvement in body image and self esteem and only minor changes in mood and distress levels. According to the researcher, the narrative documentation provided a comprehensive portrait of the women's subjective experiences of the intervention and self perceptions of its effects.

The differing results between the two data analytic approaches pose some interesting concerns regarding several components of the inquiry. Dibbell-Hope (2000) raised questions about validity or trustworthiness related to the design of both methods that might have contaminated the findings. Possible factors included: small sample; inadequate sensitivity of objective tests to measure essential features of the variables; uncontrolled differences in demographic and personal background between the different sample groups; and variances in the interpersonal dynamics of these groups.

Although the mixed methods approach failed to offer mutual support for the findings, they unmasked important methodological concerns that would not otherwise have surfaced. Likewise, this investigation clearly demonstrated the roles and significance of each method in the research process.

Dibbell-Hope's (2000) research points to how mixed methods can work in diverse ways in a project, confirming some facets, disclosing weaknesses, displaying multiple dimensions of the therapeutic process, and generating new questions. While each approach embraces different philosophical underpinnings, different constructs and design—different world views, so to speak—the sum of their parts offers a much broader and more profound perspective than could conceivably be fleshed out independently.

CONCLUSION

This chapter explored conceptual frameworks related to mixed methods research. Initially, quantitative and qualitative methods were briefly reviewed independently as were their respective overarching paradigms— deductive and inductive logic.

A point specifically underscored was that the choice of a research approach is not rooted in the superiority of one paradigm or approach over the other, but rather on contouring the model to best fit the needs of a study. This means, the mode of reasoning and research design, are subservient to and dependent upon the research questions posed. The options explored extended beyond the different research paradigms (deductive and inductive) and methods (quantitative and qualitative) to the diverse ways of mixing and matching from the smorgasbord of possibilities each affords.

Four samples of mixed methods studies (one art therapy and three dance/movement therapy) were profiled to illustrate how this framework could be applied. See Table 12-II for a summary of the mixed method samples. These examples are by no means intended to represent a comprehensive breadth of the options mixed methods afford, but rather to furnish a glimpse into the window of possibilities.

Extending the image of the child as an explorer driven by inherent curiosity and creative imagination (proposed early in this chapter), I contend that the impetus for innovation and discovery continues throughout the life span. As adults, although the paradigms and methods of inquiry remain constant, the particular phenomena studied are, most likely, far more complex and certainly more purposefully and mindfully constructed. While the child intuitively exploits all investigative possibilities, adult researchers often identify with a particular mode to the exclusion of others. Much of current research literature now veers toward an acceptance of the

Table 12-II   SUMMARY OF MIXED METHODS EXEMPLARS:
PARADIGMS AND RESEARCH DESIGNS

Researchers	Research Paradigm	Research Design(s)	Method of Data Analysis
Rehavia-Hanauer, 2003	Deductive Theory-based research question	Qualitative Case study	Qualitative Content analysis
Cruz & Hervey, 2001	Nonspecific Research question Exploratory survey	Quantitative Objective questions Qualitative Subjective questions	Quantitative Frequencies Qualitative Content analysis
Berrol, Ooi & Katz, 1997	Deductive Research question Non-directional Hypothesis	Quantitative Quasi-experimental survey Qualitative Therapists' reports, videos	Quantitative Inferential statistics Frequencies Qualitative Content analysis
Dibbell-Hope, 2000	Deductive Directional hypotheses	Quantitative Quasi-experimental Qualitative In-depth Interviews	Quantitative Inferential statistics Qualitative Content Analysis

compatibility and merits of combining methods. Such a union, when appropriate, augments the potential to build a comprehensive body of knowledge that at once presents the objective findings of the hard data and yet captures the substance and inner dynamics of the human experience in diverse societal contexts.

REFERENCES

Berrol, C. F., Ooi, W. L., & Katz, S. S. (1997). Dance/movement therapy with older adults who have sustained neurological insult: A demonstration project. *American Journal of Dance Therapy, 19*(2), 135–160.

Bloomgarten, J. (1998). Validating art therapists' tacit knowing: The heuristic experience. *Art Therapy, 15*(1), 47–50.

Borg, W. R., Gall, J. P., & Gall, M. D. (1993). *Applying educational research: a practical guide* (3rd ed.). New York: Longman.

Borg, W. R., & Gall, M. D. (1979). *Educational research: An introduction* (3rd ed.). New York: Longman.

Chodorow, J. (1991). *Dance therapy and depth psychology.* London: Routledge.

Chodorow, J. (in press). *Active imagination: Healing from within.* London: Tamu Press.

Cook, T. D., & Reichardt, C. S. (Eds.). (1979). *Qualitative and quantitative methods in evaluation research.* Beverly Hills, CA: Sage.

Cresswell, J. W. (1994). *Research design: Qualitative and quantitative approaches.* Thousand Oaks, CA: Sage.

Cruz, R. F., & Hervey, L. (2001). The American Dance Therapy Association research survey. *American Journal of Dance Therapy, 23*(2), 89–118.

Dibbell-Hope, S. (2000). The use of dance/movement therapy in psychological adaptation to breast cancer. *The Arts in Psychotherapy, 27*(1), 51–68.

Edwards, J. M. (1999). Considering the pragmatic frame: Social science research approaches relevant to research in music therapy. *The Arts in Psychotherapy, 26*(2), 73–80.

Ekman, P. (Ed.). (1998). Afterward: Universality of emotional expression? A personal history dispute. In C. Darwin, *The expression of emotions in man and animals* (3rd ed.). New York: Oxford University Press.

Forinash, M. (1995). Phenomenological research. In B. L. Wheeler (Ed.), *Music therapy research: Quantitative and qualitative perspectives* (pp. 368–387). Phoenixville, PA: Barcelona Publishers.

Gantt, L. M. (1998). A discussion of art therapy as a science. *Art Therapy, 15*(1), 3–12.

Green, J., & Horton, S. W. (1999). Postpositivist research in dance. In S. H. Fraleigh & P. Hanstein (Eds.), *Researching dance: evolving modes of inquiry* (pp. 91–123). Pittsburgh, PA: University of Pittsburgh Press.

Guralnik, D. B. (Ed.) (1992). *Webster's New World Dictionary of the American Language.* New York: Warner Brooks.

Hanstein, P. (1999a). From idea to research proposal: Balancing the systematic and serendipitous. In S. H. Fraleigh & P. Hanstein (Eds.), *Researching dance: Evolving modes of inquiry* (pp. 22–61). Pittsburgh, PA: University of Pittsburg Press.

Hanstein, P. (1999b). Models and metaphors: theory making and the creation of new knowledge. In S. H. Fraleigh & P. Hanstein (Eds.), *Researching dance: Evolving modes of inquiry* (pp. 62–90). Pittsburgh, PA: University of Pittsburgh Press.

Hedrick, T. E. (1994). The qualitative-quantitative debate: Possibilities for integration. In H. C. Reichardt & S. F. Rallis (Eds.), *The qualitative-quantitative debate: New perspective* (Vol. 61, pp. 45–52). San Francisco, CA: Jossey-Bass.

Hervey, L. (2000). *Artistic inquiry in dance/movement therapy.* Springfield, IL: Charles C Thomas.

Julliard, K. (1998). Outcome research in health care: implications for art therapy. *Art Therapy, 15*(1), 13–21.

Junge, M. B., & Linesch, D. (1993). An exploration into qualitative research in music therapy. *The Arts in Psychotherapy, 20*(1), 61–68.

Kerlinger, F. (1973). *Foundations of behavioral research* (2nd ed.). New York: Holt, Rinehart and Winston.

Lincoln, Y. S., & Guba, E. G. (1985). *Naturalistic inquiry.* Beverly Hills, CA: Sage.

McNiff, S. A. (1998). *Art-based research.* Philadelphia, PA: Jessica Kingsley.

Moustakas, C. (1994). *Phenomenological research methods.* Thousand Oaks, CA: Sage.

Neuman, I., & Benz, C. R. (1998). *Qualitative-quantitative research methodology; Exploring the interactive continuum.* Carbondale, IL: Southern Illinois University Press.

Piaget, J., & Inhelder, B. (1969). *The psychology of the child.* New York: Basic Books.

Politsky, R. H. (1995). Toward a typology of research in the creative arts therapies. *The Arts in Psychotherapy, 22*(4), 307–314.

Rehavia-Hanauer, D. (2003). Identifying conflicts of anorexia nervosa as manifested in the art therapy process. *The Arts in Psychotherapy, 30*(3), 137–149.

Reichardt, C. S., & Rallis, S. F. (1994). The quantitative-qualitative debate: New perspectives. In C. S. Reichardt, & S. F. Rallis (Eds.), *Qualitative and quantitative inquiries are not incompatible: A call for a new partnership* (Vol. 61, pp. 91–98). San Francisco, CA: Jossey-Bass Inc.

Spaniol, S. (1998). Towards an ethnographic approach to art therapy research: People with psychotic disability as collaborators. *Art Therapy, 15*(1), 29–37.

Stewart, C. T. (2001). *The symbolic impetus: How creative fantasy motivates development.* New York: Free Association Books.

Stewart, L. H. (1987). A brief report: affect and archetype. *Journal of Analytical Psychology, 32,* 35–46.

Tashakkori, A., & Teddlie, C. (1998). *Mixed methodology: Combining qualitative and quantitative approaches.* Thousand Oaks, CA: Sage.
Walizer, M. H., & Wienir, P. L. (1978). *Research methods and analysis: Searching for relationships.* New York: Harper & Row.

AUTHOR INDEX

225

SUBJECT INDEX

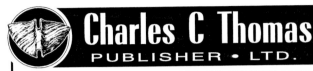

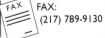
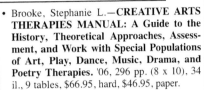
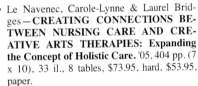